D0917015

ACTIVITIES
FOR THE
AGED AND INFIRM

Fifth Printing

ACTIVITIES

FOR THE

AGED AND INFIRM

A Handbook for the Untrained Worker

By

TONI MERRILL, M.A.

Activity Program Consultant in County Homes
Editor, the Oldster
Division of Public Assistance
Department of Public Welfare in Wisconsin
Madison, Wisconsin

With a Foreword By

LOIS J. HARDT, Ph.D.
Program Consultant,
National Society for Crippled Children and Adults, Inc.
Chicago, Illinois

Drawings by

HAZEL McCLAIN

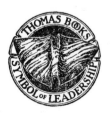

CHARLES C THOMAS • PUBLISHER
Springfield • Illinois • U.S.A.

Published and Distributed Throughout the World by
CHARLES C THOMAS • PUBLISHER
BANNERSTONE HOUSE
301-327 East Lawrence Avenue, Springfield, Illinois, U.S.A.

© *1967 by* CHARLES C THOMAS • PUBLISHER
ISBN 0-398-01294-6
Library of Congress Catalog Card Number: 66-24635

First Printing, 1967
Second Printing, 1969
Third Printing, 1972
Fourth Printing, 1975
Fifth Printing, 1977

With THOMAS BOOKS *careful attention is given to all details of*
manufacturing and design. It is the Publisher's desire to present
books that are satisfactory as to their physical qualities and artistic
possibilities and appropriate for their particular use. THOMAS
BOOKS *will be true to those laws of quality that assure a good name*
and good will.

Printed in the United States of America
N-1

Dedicated

to the good people who care for the
aged and infirm in Wisconsin county homes

FOREWORD

The MODERN concept of dynamic rehabilitation of the ill and impaired has validity and application in caring for the aged and infirm. The "team approach" of coordinated, inter-disciplinary procedure is being put into practice in ever-increasing numbers of institutions and programs for the elderly and chronically disabled. Today the "poor farms" and "asylums" which offered static custodial care are being replaced by institutions of the highest calibre, which give not only care, but which actively endeavor to at least maintain and often to regain the highest level of function for the individual residents.

Unfortunately, the paramedical services which accompany the medical aspects of modern rehabilitation are very costly, and when the administrator must work with limited financial resources, he is forced to either forego or diminish those services which appear to have the least tangible and measurable results.

The service called "recreation" is one of these, and although the detrimental effects of social isolation and idleness have been fully recognized, the values of recreational experiences as combatants of this deterioration have not been fully recognized.

Perhaps the values have never fully perceived because the potential of recreation and socialization has never been fully exploited and realized. For too long a time, the adjunctive therapy of recreation and socialization was relegated to an existence dependent upon the "Lady Bountifuls" who allied themselves with the institution. Untrained, given no leadership, no equipment, no budget and no meaningful time in the daily schedule, the well-meaning and dedicated volunteers evolved the only program they knew — they did **for** rather than **with** — and for many years, the passive entertainment type of recreation and socialization which these volunteers provided were the only bright spots in the long days of the institution residents.

Just as we have come to recognize that maximum rehabilitation

vii

or the maximum maintenance of habitation can only be achieved through a process of combined efforts of medical and paramedical disciplines, we also realize that each contributing discipline must be equally dynamic and aggressive. The socio-recreational phase of the procedure, therefore, cannot be static or passive and still make its contribution to the process. But even as we recognize this, we lack sufficient trained professional recreation personnel to direct the socialization aspect, and we probably never will have adequate personnel to do all that could be done.

We have needed, therefore, and we shall always need, the volunteers, the untrained but dedicated people who fill the personnel and program void by giving long hours of untiring effort; and we, the professionals, must aid and enhance their efforts by providing them with the tools to carry out our programs.

This book is a tool. Written by a professional for the volunteer, it tells why, how, what, when and where. It shows the way to do **with** rather than merely **for**. In using this book, the reader will not only find step-by-step directions and methods, but will also read of the creativity of other volunteers and hopefully be encouraged to create anew.

L. J. HARDT, PH.D.

PREFACE

THIS BOOK IS DESIGNED for people interested in the care of the increasing numbers of residents[1] in nursing homes, private homes or patients in hospitals, and for people who have the responsibility for organizing and conducting appropriate programs to reach them.

It consists of an exchange of ideas, procedures, and aids from forty-four recreation programs in Wisconsin county homes, county general hospitals and volunteer programs sponsored by a variety of public and private agencies, organizations and community groups.

One function of the leader is to perform with minimal guidance in general activity and supportive or maintenance programs, providing something for all residents. A common understanding of goals should be reached by those in position to direct and influence the program: "To provide opportunities for all residents to participate at their optimum levels of function; to maintain the physical, social, and emotional functioning of residents at its highest level."[2]

Nearly everyone is concerned, puzzled or burdened with the responsibilities of caring for an aged or handicapped relative or friend; the nursing home resident himself is distressed by his inadequacies, depressed by his dependence on others and often apologetic about the care he requires.

One must then, develop programs which come to the resident on the wards and in his room, to which he is not only invited but is actually urged. Activities described in this book can be enjoyed by everyone of every age and inclination, but they were selected because of their particular suitability for specific limitations.

---

[1] The book refers to nursing home "residents"; although if they require maximum nursing care, they are referred to as "patients."

[2] Marilyn Hennessy, OTR, Chronic Disease and Aging, Wisconsin State Board of Health.

"How-to-do" is needed by those who care — their families, recreational and group workers, educators and religious leaders, welfare workers, nurses, nursing home administrators, volunteers — indeed, the disabled or handicapped themselves.

Activities for the Aged and Infirm hopefully can be used as a manual, a do-it-yourself kit to read and follow step by step, although the leader needs to draw also on ideas from every experience in life: in every book he reads, every walk around the square, any article in the local newspaper or an evening TV show.

TONI MERRILL, M.A.

ACKNOWLEDGMENTS

THE AUTHOR IS indebted in a large part for editing, commentaries and countless suggestions in content, organization, and wording to L. J. Hardt, Ph.D. While this book has been prepared, Dr. Hardt has been the assistant professor of education in the field of rehabilitative recreation at the University of Wisconsin, and is now program consultant with the National Society of Crippled Children and Adults (the National Easter Seal Society), Chicago, Illinois.

Other grateful acknowledgments go to Miss Marilyn Hennessy, OTR, Occupational Therapy Consultant, Division of Chronic Disease and Aging, Wisconsin State Board of Health, for making valuable suggestions and corrections in rough copy revisions.

Further appreciation is expressed to Mr. William McNown, also in the Division of Public Assistance, Wisconsin Department of Public Welfare, and to Mrs. Ruth Swenson of the Wisconsin Library Commission.

The great bulk of the script has been assembled from experiences in county home visits, where activity programs have been developed by the activity aides, OTR's and COTA's or other county home employees or volunteers working in these areas who have been resourceful and original in expanding programs with new ideas, giving variety and color to geriatric activities.

T. M.

Work, some activity, playing at a favorite hobby, should continue for as long as a person lives and breathes. Activity and keeping occupied is one of the "staffs of life." We decline when we have no interests, nothing to work for.

Grandma Moses, you've had a full, productive life. Do you have a message for people in their seventy's or older that may help them enjoy their remaining years more?

I don't know how much good it will do, but I would tell them not to think about growing old or dying. The Lord put us on this earth to enjoy ourselves, and we should. They will be happier if they forget about their age and think about helping others.

*Parade. Parade Publications Inc., 1961, 733 Third Avenue, New York.

CONTENTS

PART I

PERSONNEL AND PLANNING

PART II

GAMES AND ACTIVITIES FOR OLDSTERS

PART III

SPECIAL PARTIES AND QUIZZES FOR ALL RESIDENTS

ACTIVITIES
FOR THE
AGED AND INFIRM

PART I

PERSONNEL AND PLANNING

Chapter I

THE LEADER

Their smiles, their love, is my reward.

Who Is The Leader?

IN THIS BOOK the employee in charge of the program is referred to as an "activity aide"; that is, a director of the programs (many of whom may have been attendants on the wards) appointed by the superintendent to be responsible for the "activity program"; sometimes it is a registered occupational therapist working full time or part time, or a certified occupational therapy assistant (COTA) trained in geriatrics. Sometimes it must be the assistant superintendent or a responsible volunteer.

The leader is friendly, warm, understanding and accepts others; he is familiar with oldsters' backgrounds — religious, social, occupational and educational — and respects their views. Patient in disposition, a successful activity aide will try to be relaxed, even-tempered and won't attempt to rush the handicapped, confused or senescent oldster. Tactful and just, he can smooth over the ruffled feelings, likes fun and is willing to laugh at himself. Open-minded and resourceful, he has initiative and is willing to try new ideas. Kind, without showing pity, he feels empathy.

A leader who likes the aged and infirm is resourceful, a good organizer and is adaptable, kind and tactful — sometimes he also has skills in handicrafts, music or other activities.

In some states, consulting services are available and some training and recommendations may be requested. Because the activity aide is limited in skills doesn't mean he can't expand a program by learning other skills. He must be willing to recognize his limitations and be willing and able to recruit volunteers who are often expert and experienced in other activity projects which will reach more residents.

In leadership, the leader creates a situation in which people believe in him to the extent that they willingly work for and with his ideas. An understanding leader gives residents what they think they want and makes them want what they should have.

"Strategies of Leadership" and "Leadership Techniques for a Single Event" are merely guides with built-in goals for which to strive. They embrace leadership in all fields of recreation activity, and it is up to activity leader in the nursing home setting to adapt these qualifications to his own use. If the reader sees a reference which is not applicable to his situation (i.e., "Are the leader's responsibilities related to his training?"), he must not think, "This isn't applicable to me since I'm an untrained volunteer." Some understanding and application of use to the Home, the program, the residents and the leader must go with this material.

Steps for the Leader

1. **Seek administrative decision and approval to develop an activity program in the Home[1] or hospital.**

2. **Make a survey of the areas** in the Home where activities could be held — the patio, the porch, the living room, recreation room, chapel, dining room, solarium, park or lawn areas.

3. **Decide on a monthly budget,** no matter how limited; an amount on which to depend. Programs must of necessity rely on salvage materials, donations and inexpensive items; but the leader determines an amount — five dollars or ten dollars — for crepe paper; nail polish for the charm glass; glue, pencils, scissors, construction paper, etc., by determining the number of residents to be reached, how often they will be reached in a given period, which activities will be used and which will need supplies, and estimating the amount of material each resident in each activity will use.

4. **Find something for everyone:** Even the most handicapped and the bedridden may like visitors scheduled regularly with a simple craft or game. From the suggestions of the resident himself and from staff members, the aide lists activities to be tried.

---

[1] In this book, the word **Home,** written with a capital H, refers to an institution for the elderly rather than a domicile.

Strategies of Leadership[2]

1. Be enthusiastic and show it; smile, have fun and keep a laugh in your voice. People will take their cues from you.

2. Never embarrass anyone. This implies that activities should be easy; skillful performance is relatively unimportant; minor mistakes are overlooked, and games are avoided in which some have fun at the expense of others. Be patient, helpful, sympathetic and kind. Relax, be human and let your sense of humor show. It has been aptly said that a good social recreation leader "is limber, loving and a little bit loony."

3. Know your activities and be skilled in their presentation. Confidence is based on knowledge and skill. In general, these steps should be followed in introducing a new game:

   a. Place the group in formation.
   b. Name the game.
   c. Explain it briefly; avoid long, drawn-out explanations.
   d. Demonstrate it, if necessary.
   e. Ask for questions.
   f. Start immediately.
   g. Observe play carefully and make whatever changes are necessary to improve it.
   h. Encourage players or teams verbally.
   i. Stop play before interest begins to lag and introduce a new activity.

4. Adapt the activity to the ability level of the group. For example, a game or relay may involve running if youths are taking part, but should be changed to walking if women in high-heeled shoes are playing. Also, be prepared to adjust to conditions and situations you were unable to foresee, such as variation in the number of participants anticipated or a lack of game supplies.

5. Use a whistle sparingly, if at all. It is best to use it only as a signal for the group to become quiet so instructions may be given. When it is used for more than one purpose, the

---

[2] Howard Danford: **Creative Leadership in Recreation.** Boston, Allyn and Bacon, 1954, pp. 153-154. Material is being quoted by permission of publisher.

group frequently is confused since it can't tell for which purpose it is blown.

6. Stand where you can be seen and speak so you can be heard. Act in a confident manner. Any evidence of a lack of confidence on your part will quickly be sensed by the group and will constitute a major handicap. Never try to outtalk an inattentive group. Secure attention by a short, sharp blast on your whistle, raising your hand or just standing quietly.

7. Never choose up sides because of the embarrassment to those chosen last. Use some impersonal method of dividing into teams.

8. If awards (or prizes) are presented, they should be inexpensive.

9. Use words that people understand and supplement verbal instructions with gestures when desirable. For example, when you instruct a group to move in a counterclockwise direction indicate what you mean by a sweeping movement of the arm. Also, raise your voice at the end of a sentence when you wish to stimulate action; in starting a contest or relay say, "Ready — go!"

10. Dress appropriately for the occasion. What is appropriate depends upon such factors as the nature of the event, its location, the group and even the day. When in doubt you would do well to lean toward conservatism.

Leadership Techniques for a Single Event[3]

The following techniques are important to the leader of a social event and can be mastered by volunteer leaders interested in effective leadership. The competent leader:

1. Knows what he is going to say and do before coming before the group. He is prepared.

2. Speaks clearly and distinctly. He speaks as though he expects the group to listen, and they usually will.

3. Is in a position where all the group can see and hear him.

---

[3] The Recreation Program. Chicago, The Athletic Institute, 1963, p. 315-16. By special permission from the publisher.

4. Secures the attention of the group before starting an event by raising his hand, blowing a whistle, breaking a balloon or speaking quietly until the group quiets down.

5. Demonstrates as well as describes an activity but believes individuals have "fun in doing" so he gets them into the activity quickly.

6. Establishes rapport at this first appearance. This is often done by a story, a joke, or with an event which captures attention and sets the tone of the event.

7. Develops and works his plan but is still flexible and willing to modify his plan to fit the mood and tempo of the occasion. He has more events planned than he will need. This gives him confidence.

8. Does not have fun at another's expense; does not exploit another's gullibility. It is just as much fun to use a willing, but wise, stooge.

9. Keeps the group playing. He avoids activities in which there are too many dropouts, or games in which too few are occupied. If he chooses an event that involves only a few, he makes sure it has entertainment value for the spectators.

10. Does not choose sides for he knows how it feels to be the last one chosen. He uses some automatic and impersonal device for dividing the groups.

11. Saves time by avoiding awkward shifts from one formation to another. He works out a sequence so that games requiring the same formation are bracketed and so that shifts from one game to another involve the least change and movement.

12. Uses assistants. If an activity is at all complicated and calls for instruction, he trains a team of helpers in advance and distributes them among the group.

13. Rehearses. After planning the program, he gives it a trial run working out unsatisfactory parts and anticipating all possible situations. Rehearsals can be as much fun for the committee as the party itself.

14. Is ready. He avoids fumbling, stalling and indecision by jotting down his order of events on handy-sized cards. He

believes the group will follow the leader who knows where he is going.

15. Stops the activity while it still has zest, while the group still wants to play it, knowing that he can use it again and that the group will not be too fatigued or disinterested in the next activity.

16. Has an ending. He has a decisive ending to a social event. He believes a short social event is preferable to one which is artificially drawn out. He ends with a strong finale.

The Leader's Schedule

The administrator and perhaps the nurse, or whoever needs to know his whereabouts, should have the activity aide's schedule, which he draws up with his supervisor's approval.

(Home and Infirmary Activity Program)

Monday — 9-10:30 AM   Men of Home and infirmary in crafts.
1:30-3 PM   Games in chapel area, Home and infirmary.

Tuesday —   AM   All floors of infirmary 2-3-4, people mentally alert.
1:30-3 PM   *Weekly Reader*, Home and infirmary chapel area.

Wednesday —   AM   Crafts and games in Home one week, cooking class alternate weeks.
PM   Activities in chapel area — cards, games, conversation, music.

Thursday —   AM   All floors in infirmary in crafts 2-3-4.
PM   Men of Home and infirmary in crafts.

Friday —   AM   Home ladies in activity center.
PM   Open for special people who work with special programs, weaving, talent shows.

Daily

7:45-9 AM   Staff conference.
Preparation.
9-10:30 AM   Escorting patients to activity area, conducting activity.

10:30 AM - 1:30 PM	Escorting patients back to floors. Putting materials away. Lunch.
1:30-3 PM	Preparation and conducting activity. Records; individual residents' records are filled out.
3-4 PM	Escorting patients back to floors. Putting materials away. Cleaning up. Records filled out. Conference with superior.

Chapter II

THE RESIDENT

* Never underestimate the power of the human spirit.

IDENTIFYING THE POPULATION IN THE HOME

BECAUSE OF THEIR emotional status as well as their being physically ill, residents are hard to care for: nursing care requires time and costly treatment. Good leadership in an activity aide can result in better care for residents at a financial saving for them and for the administrator of the Home and hospital.

Besides residents' physical infirmities, one must also know their emotional make-up — the depressed, the withdrawn, the cantankerous and the hypersensitive. Knowing something of their life history, their economic disapppointments and their physical discouragements, enables one to better understand their emotional ills.

With many, the spouse has died and all the children are gone; sometimes there is no correspondence, and no one knows they are in the Home. Many residents who feel themselves to be a burden on the world say, "I've spent all my life working, scrimping, and saving, and now see where I am! Isn't this terrible?"

The aged and infirm are generally people who have lived good lives, who have worked hard making a living; they have raised families and have been good citizens. They feel disgraced by needing financial aid; they miss the room at home, the house and garden on a familiar street, neighbors and familiar faces they once knew. Sometimes they say, "I pray each day that I may die in the night."

Doctors and nurses have made it possible for hearts to continue beating, sometimes when almost everything else in the bodies have given out. Sometimes, in a new nursing home, men in over-

---

* From the movie "Proud Years." Center for Mass Communication of Columbia University Press, 1125 Amsterdam Avenue, New York, N.Y.

alls just sit although everything in the room is new: the bed, the dresser, the chair; but here they are with their hands in their laps. Their hands and feet are capable of performing; good eyes and hearing are still theirs, yet they feel lonely and a little frightened.

The Home is set up to give good nursing care; everything will be clean and efficient, the meals well balanced and well prepared; the rooms will be warm and they will be cared for; but will there be anyone who will care if they are there or not? Will there be anyone who has time to talk or to sit and listen?

Are they to spend their years walking around unfamiliar rooms, up and down the hall and back again? Are they too old and discouraged to make any friends, to be useful and needed as everyone needs to be?

What do the aged and infirm want to do? What can they do? What opportunities for enjoying life and filling their needs are available to them? To what kinds of recreational activities and interests do they most willingly respond? What type of group and community participation will give them greater personal satisfaction, self-confidence and status? How can the right kinds of recreation be provided for the handicapped and disabled?

How do they feel about hobbies, about fun? Sometimes they bristle and say, "I never played cards; I'm not going to start now." Many aged people who think of work as a virtue think of fun as a vice. They have spent their lives working hard and have never had time for "hobbies" or special interests; sometimes their religion opposes certain activities; language handicaps must be considered. The activity aide interviews each resident and finds his interests; he posts the list on the bulletin board for visitors, staff and volunteers to see. Observations and talks with the resident help discover program ideas.

Among the aged and infirm, their many needs are the same as those of all other human beings:

> Need to love and the opportunity to express affection.
> Need to be respected and to feel actually needed.
> Need to participate in groups, to be useful, to belong.
> Need to accept and discharge responsibilities.

Need to look forward to new friends and tasks.
Need to have creative experience.
Need to seek spiritual aid.

Superintendents, nurses, therapists and doctors aware of the problem of patients' low morale as well as the financial burden of bed care, have insisted on getting patients up and dressed at least part of the day, unless they are critically ill. The old notion of leaving the patients alone in rocking chairs to drowse, to weep or to quarrel has been turned into an invitation to take part in some form of a game or a visit from a friend, perhaps folding bandages or working on a quilt.

Chapter III

THE PROGRAM

We do more for ourselves and more for one another.

PLANNING THE PROGRAM

THE AGED and infirm are adults, not children. To talk down to them, to belittle them, to imply by an inflection of the voice that they are less than adults is to insult, embarrass, and hurt. To infer that "they are in their second childhood" does them a great deal of harm, since by doing so one makes them **dependent,** rather than **strengthening them to independency,** the goal in rehabilitation. One must approach them as adults.

Among the principles of motivation, one might list the resident's background, studying his special interest questionnaire, establishing friendly relationships with him, making conversations with him free and easy and warm.

The resident interview can be a revelation; armed with paper and pencil the activity aide visits each of the rooms in the Home or hospital, introduces himself, asks the resident's name, visits and takes notes. If the resident is a man, can he do carpentry, sand breadboards, repair toys for children, play cards, learn weaving, join a discussion class? If the resident is a woman, can she knit, tat, crochet, sew, would she enjoy singing, like to belong to a Ladies Aid in the Home? Does she have other suggestions? Rides? Stuffing animals and dolls for children in the community?

The things that seem to appeal most are things residents can do for others. "What is it for?" they want to know. "Who'll use is? What good is it?" One indicates in conversation the need for the resident being interviewed and what he or she can produce, how it may improve him physically and how he might enjoy it. Often the resident says he used to play checkers or some other game which may mean that he would play with some help and encouragement. If he says, "I liked playing cards, but I haven't played for years," the aide produces a card holder, sits down and plays a game with him, if the aide knows how; if not, he produces someone — another resident or a volunteer — who does.

If the resident is visually handicapped, the activity aide orders a special game for the blind. If a woman indicates that she at one time crocheted but now has arthritic fingers, perhaps the aide brings out a large set of wooden crochet hooks; instead of just talking about it, the aide starts an activity on the spot.

Patient Interest Sheets

The patient interest sheet may be filled out by anyone intending to follow through with it as far as residents' activities are concerned. After the sheet is compiled, it should be at hand for the person who will use it, whether it be contacting the resident personally to invite him to each of the interest-activities checked, making as many activities available as possible, or referring his interest to a volunteer capable of carrying it out.

Perhaps introducing the resident to other residents who will share the game, the hobby or craft will suffice to promote it. Frequent checks should be made to see that he has been invited to participate in as many interests as possible, or the reason discovered as to why he has not participated, if this is the case. The sheet ought to be dated and reviewed to be updated whenever interest lags appreciably.

SCOPE AND OBJECTIVES

Program goals must be centered on the resident's needs, not on what the leader enjoys doing most. Focusing on the residents' needs, interests and potentials, one starts the program plans.

A program of variety should be relaxing and stimulating, active and passive, individual and group, inside the Home and outside in the community.

The leader should consider the accessibility of the Home to the community, the age and health of the resident and the effect of the program on him; he should see that the activities meet

TABLE I
INDIVIDUAL RESIDENT'S PROGRAM REPORT

Resident's Name

Activities Report

1. Home Newspaper (or other writing projects):

   Mildly Interested   _Actively Interested_   _Excellent Participation_

2. Discussion Group:

   Mildly Interested   _Actively Interested_   _Excellent Participation_

3. Work Assignments:

   Mildly Interested   _Actively Interested_   _Excellent Participation_

4. Musical Groups:

   Mildly Interested   _Actively Interested_   _Excellent Participation_

5. New Table Games (or renewed activity with old familiar games):

   Mildly Interested   _Actively Interested_   _Excellent Participation_

6. Social Clubs and Parties:

   Mildly Interested   _Actively Interested_   _Excellent Participation_

7. Resident Council:

   Mildly Interested   _Actively Interested_   _Excellent Participation_

8. Exercise Group:

   Mildly Interested   _Actively Interested_   _Excellent Participation_

9. Gardening, Rides, Walks, Outside Activities:

   Mildly Interested   _Actively Interested_   _Excellent Participation_

10. Carpentry, Arts and Crafts:

    Mildly Interested   _Actively Interested_   _Excellent Participation_

Improvements: Social Relationships

                Physical Benefits

Other Comments:

                                Activity Aide

TABLE II

FORM PRESENTED TO THE RESIDENT AT THE TIME OF ADMISSION

Welcome Wagon

Recreation Office — Ext. 238

Information Office — Ext. 844

Green House — Ext. 110

Recreation Hall Hours:

Monday - Friday   8 A.M. - 4 P.M.

Sunday Services   9:30 A.M.

Craft Shop   8 A.M. - 4 P.M.

Hello:

    We would like to "clue you in" on the Home activity facilities available for your use. The map shows you where we are located.

    We want your ideas, too, for things you'd like to do. We can't use ideas that are castles in the air but we will welcome some workable suggestions. Thanks for your help!

In Your Ward (with medical approval)

1. Individual card and box games.
2. Hobby and special interest groups.
3. Piano and song sheets.
4. Radios.
5. Red Cross visits and shopping.
6. Entertainment by community groups.
7. Parties sponsored by community groups.

Your activity aide's name is

....

Your social worker's name is

....

In the Home Building

1. Pool Room.
2. Craft Room.
3. Cards and other table games.
4. Bingo (Saturday evenings).
5. Monthly hostess party.
6. Planned evening recreation.
7. Trips (see aide).
8. Musical facilities:
   a. Phonographs and records.
   b. Piano and music.
9. TV Room.
10. Beauty Shop and Barber Shop.

Cordially,

Activity Staff

Information

Date ....

Name .... Ward ....

1. Birthday? ....
2. What town are you from? ....
   ....
3. Hobbies? ....
4. Favorite card games? ....
   ....

5. Favorite indoor recreation? ....
   ....
6. What types of music do you enjoy?
   ....
7. What types of entertainment do you like? ....

Your Suggestions or Requests:

TABLE III

PATIENT INTEREST SHEET

Name: ....Room # .... Date of Birth ....

Family: ....Religion ....

Physical Limitations ....

....

Special Need: ....

Interests:

Frame Weaving .... Sewing .... Knitting ....
Rug Weaving .... Crocheting .... Embroidery ....

ART: Water Color .... Finger Paint .... Ceramics .... Oil ....
Drawing .... Clay Modeling .... Decorations ....

Leather Craft .... Wood Work .... Mosaic Tile .... Copper ....
Books .... Music .... Singing .... Instruments ....
Newspaper .... Dry Floral Arranging .... Photography ....
Stamps .... Sports .... Cooking ....
TV .... Movies .... Hobby ....

Games: Cards.......... Checkers.......... Monopoly.......... Chinese Checkers..........
Chess .... Cross Word Puzzles .... Quizzes ....
Cribbage .... Shuffleboard .... Dominoes .... Poker ....
Bingo .... Pokeno .... Bowling ....

Additional Interests or Comments:

the needs and interests of the participant and the cultural and ethnic coloring of his background in planning the program.

Social activities may come in many forms from birthday parties to social clubs or ward contests. Entertainment has many values: residents enjoy seeing new faces and making new friends. Programs by local groups can be easily arranged, are inexpensive or cost nothing and usually mean good public relations. The disasters of "outside entertainment" sometimes result from poor planning between the Home and the volunteers; sometimes a program is unsuited and uninteresting to the age group and not always well spaced in time — too many in December and too few in January, for instance.

It's wrong to accept just any entertainment that comes along — the leader should be selective, the plan well discussed with the superintendent and volunteers, the acceptable features considered and full explanation given as to why some of it would not be acceptable to the Home.

In democratic procedure, the leader forms a council that meets regularly, with residents and staff represented. Sources could be a suggestion box, visiting with the resident, calling on the community for help in community programs, religious services or volunteers in a wide source of programs giving variety and establishing community good will.

The leader assumes that a variety of spectator activities finds its way into the Home — movies, TV and other entertainment, and is more concerned with the really hard part of the job, that of "activating the resident." This doesn't happen easily; since there are never any dramatic starts in a geriatric program, one works slowly, day by day, beginning happily with a few who are interested, perhaps around a table.

Recreation programs in the nursing homes and hospitals have come to mean more than just leisure-time-filling activities; more and more stress is given self-help, rehabilitating the resident to do more for himself and more for one another. If he can keep his fingers active playing dominoes or Chinese checkers, he can continue to feed himself. He can play horseshoes, beanbags, bowl from a wheelchair, keep his arm in motion, join a team where he makes friends, learn to laugh and slap a friend on the back, even if his score is poor.

Hopefully, the Homes will keep individual records of residents' activities on a daily or weekly basis which take only a few minutes a day but help as a yardstick toward a more complete recreation program.

The aide asks as he works, "What is this activity doing for the resident — does it fill any of his needs? Does it give him self respect, a feeling of being useful, of making new friends, of learning something?"

Because he works with people's physical disabilities and limitations, he asks, "What is he physically able to do? Is he a bed patient, senescent, in a wheelchair, able to use his hands, able to see; is he musically inclined or is he ambulatory?"

Categorized activities in this book may suggest activities which will fill the needs.

Ways of reaching the needs of the resident (each one who is, of course, an individual and each one different) are limitless. With each physical improvement, one tries more activity in social groups, educational clubs, music, Friendly Visitors, physical exercise, intellectual stimulation, social interrelation, creative expression and spectator appreciation.

Goals of a program are met: reaching the hard-to-reach; each leader seeks them out with his own special personal appeal.

Motivation

Motivating the aged and infirm into activity isn't always easy—one hears them say, "I've worked all my life," "I'm tired," "I can't get out of this wheelchair," or "I can't leave my room," "I have no one who cares," "I wish I could die," "Noise bothers me," "I never played games."

The programs must be directed and supervised to give permanence and importance. Games and equipment won't be used unless there are leaders — employed or volunteer — to schedule the activity and invite the residents to play; and then they'll get up out of chairs to join a group, taking part in an activity with someone.

Often rules of a game must be quickly adjusted to the limitations of certain members of the group to encourage them, changing the distances or handicapping others in the game, for instance, giving the resident less distance to throw the ball or asking the more able to use his left hand in some physical competition.

Despite the discouragements the leader bravely labors, often with many appeals reaching even the hard to reach:

We showed them the attractive samples, and before long they were making quilts. Volunteers brought yarn and material backing. We received a letter of thanks from a mother of thirteen, a mother who wanted to come and visit the Home. Sometimes one resident can motivate others better than we can. Giving instead of receiving is a connecting link with others in the community who aren't aware of our Home or what it is doing.

One teaches him to take on responsibility for organizing play or work like taking care of scrapbooks of world events. Giving him an idea of what he can do, the aide says she'll be coming back at such and such a time, makes two or three suggestions, gay and happy about what he's able to do since he wants appreciation and responds to encouragement.

Working individually with those who don't understand, we try to increase their mental alertness and not let them get too far away from the world, increasing feelings of achievement.

When Arella came as an eighty-year-old polio victim, I learned about her through her pastor. I wish you could have seen some of the wonderful things she's done since we got her interested in cross-stitch embroidery. We got a walker for her and "bragged" her up on how independent she had become. We said, "When you can walk to the dining room, we'll move you to ground floor." All of a sudden she said, "I don't want this walker any more." We put it in the storeroom, and there it's been. Because she had been a teacher, we said, "What did you teach your pupils? You practice the same thing you taught them." She said, "My mother was ashamed of me because I had a crippled hand." In her eighties, she's improving all the time. She took a bus last month to a wedding in Minneapolis, going to a strange city all by herself.

"My fingers are stiff," they say, but we find easy jobs for them, like making cork coasters, cut and ready to assemble. As soon as we show them how easy it is, they will do it. As soon as they say, "I couldn't possibly do that," we tell them to watch; then they say, "Do you suppose I could do it?"

It's better if we have men and women together. Also, an adoption system is good, with residents and volunteers. One man had been here since 1937 with no further correspondence and needed a friend. We pick someone who is overly-communicative, and he'll soon get the hard-to-reach motivated.

Don't you find your coffee pot has been one of your best friends in motivating residents? In getting them down for the first time, this is an excellent thing.

We call them Cleopatra and Lady Astor and Mrs. Vanderbilt — they all have names for themselves after permanents and facials. We find this is a good way to get women motivated into other activities once they have become interested in their appearance again.

We found if we interview the resident as soon as he comes in, it's a help. So many times people come in — maybe they have kept house, tried to live with children — and they don't know what to do with themselves. We start immediately to let them know we're here and interested.

Olga has had a nervous breakdown and has been just blank until her family told us she used to love playing bingo, but she didn't respond. Her daughter had brought a weaving set, but she paid no attention and the aides had to tell her to say good-bye to her daughter when she left; we almost had to take her to bingo bodily. We played several games with her just watching, but finally she found the numbers by herself. Physically she's in good health, but we feel hopeful that a little game like bingo may have started a new life for her in the Home.

The volunteers asked one another, "What can we give Elmer?" He's handicapped so that he uses just one hand, and is also mentally retarded to some extent, but they found a toy car for him to push across the table in front of him in a game; and he used his hand and arm for the first time, and is gaining more strength all the time.

Sarah would throw a tantrum like a child, a pseudo-seizure. Through ignoring this and through gentle persuasion we urged her to make stuffed dolls and dress them. She decorated pumpkins with painted faces and hats a few months ago.

John refused and refused and refused to be interested in an activity, but we kept asking him, until we finally got John in. We try not to miss anyone. They like to do something for others, and our men like crafts more than women. A great many of our people who can't use their hands, prefer games. One of them was motivated by sorting jewelry that was usable for prizes or for decorations.

Love and recognition are important in dealing with residents. One ought to treat the oldster as an individual who has a great need for love. It's important for the worker to be cheerful and gay, even though she may not be up to par that day. The leader is here to help the resident and shouldn't burden him with other troubles. She ought to increase interaction on working and playing together and sit down and talk with the patient, and eventually another resident will feel left out and will want to join the group at the table.

Sometimes the resident says, "Why should I do that now? I didn't do that when I was a kid." But the staff keeps him interested, keeps him in contact with others, gets him to work with others and to know one another, lets everyone participate, no matter how little, and has him help others, which is something he wants.

We must have something that interests men, the blind residents, the hard-to-reach. In motivation, we must find something they are able to do.

I take a basket of craft supplies — crochet and embroidery cotton and yarn — and sit down and visit at their bedsides and soon they are involved in a craft. I interview residents as to what they would like to do. They love the attention, and it's an "in."

Chapter IV

FACILITIES

The place: for companionship, for expressing oneself, for achieving status, for play and fun, for occupying free time, for learning new skills, for "showing someone how," for feeling a part of a team.

THE AREAS IN WHICH TO WORK

ANOTHER aspect to consider in planning the program is the size of the room in which to work. There must be a place for people to sit down, room for wheelchairs and tables, a place for some supplies to be used even though limited, adequate lighting for craft work or reading, tables high enough for the wheelchairs, room temperature suitable for the activity, and an area near the bathrooms. Perhaps the best place to start is with a small group around the table in the solarium or in the living room on their floor; transporting wheelchairs down elevators is slow and laborious.

To furnish and supply these areas with proper equipment and supplies, Homes often rely on a philanthropic organization, relatives and friends who want to give a gift in memorial, or financially able volunteers. Home leaders post a list of needed equipment approved by the administrator in the bulletin boards or print it occasionally in the auxiliary newsletter so that volunteers may know what is needed and how the supply or equipment will be used by residents in making a better program possible. Thus when the inquiry is made, "How can I help?" a specific answer is immediately available.

PROPER EQUIPMENT

The following list of equipment for Homes for the aged is

---

[1] Morton Thompson, Ed. D., Director, Consulting Service on Recreation for the Ill and Handicapped, National Recreation and Park Association.

suggested: National Recreation and Park Association's Consulting Service on Recreation for the Ill and Handicapped. It is not all-inclusive but can be supplemented by the specific needs of a particular Home and by the interests and backgrounds of the residents. This list may seem extensive and expensive but one doesn't have to have all of it prior to starting a program.

Basic Equipment

Equipment cart (for games, crafts, books and magazines for bedridden patients)

> Portable blackboard.
> Books and magazines.
> Quiet games (cards, checkers, chips, Scrabble®, lotto, anagrams, puzzles, Chinese checkers, dominoes).
> Active games (ring toss, suction darts, beanbag toss, shuffleboard, croquet, rubber horseshoes).
> Diversional arts crafts (painting, leather work, looms, sewing, knitting, crocheting material, paste, construction paper, drawing materials).
> Tool kit (for residents' use in construction hobbies).
> Wheel chair tables.
> Card tables.
> Card holders.
> Oversized cards (for poor eyes).

Music Equipment

> Portable organ or moveable piano.
> TV sets.
> Phonograph variable speed.
> Records (old-time songs and songs related to the basic cultural background of the group).
> Rhythm band instruments.

Movie Equipment

> Projector (16 mm).
> Slide projector.
> Screen.

Outdoor Equipment

Barbecue grill.
Aluminum tables and chairs or benches.
Deck chairs, chaise lounges.
Umbrellas.
Garden tools.
Outdoor games equipment (quoits, horseshoes, shuffleboard).

Chapter V

RECORDS AND REPORTS

°There's no satisfaction in life like being useful.

Scheduling the Program

THE ADMINISTRATOR, nurse and activity aide sit down together and discuss each activity before it's scheduled, jotting down goals for the activity: In what ways will it be useful to the resident? What area should be used for the activity and what supplies and equipment, no matter how minor, will be needed? How will these be acquired? When will the activity be scheduled? By working around other important schedules like doctor's rounds, naps, baths and visiting hours, schedules for the activity program are set up during the hours the residents can be reached.

The program schedule may be posted on a large calendar on a bulletin board in the activity room, at the nurses' station, in the elevator at wheelchair height, or in the superintendent's office and printed in the Home newspaper. Residents and staff want to know where to find it any time. Often special announcements are made over the PA system just before the activity, as reminders to residents and staff.

Activity Program Reports

Submitted to the administrator or superintendent at the end of the month, simple records notify him at a glance what's happening in activity program progress; often he needs a report to show his trustees that their investment in the activity aide's salary and supply costs are justified. Sometimes the activity aide adds a paragraph listing new activities introduced that month,

---

° From the movie "Proud Years." Center for Mass Communication of Columbia University Press, 1125 Amsterdam Avenue, New York, N.Y.

TABLE IV

WEEKLY ACTIVITY PROGRAM FOR THE AGED AND INFIRM

(Set upon a weekly basis, each activity an hour in length,
one chooses a week and sets up a program)

Monday	Tuesday	Wednesday	Thursday	Friday
9:30 AM Domino Tournament 1:30 Music Appreciation Class 2:30 Residents' Planning Committee for Home Newspaper	9:30 AM Green Thumb Club 1:30 If You Like to Sing, Join the Choral Group 2:30 Committee to Decorate the Home for the Month	9:30 AM Program Committee Meets 1:30 Card Party 2:30 Craft Group	9:30 AM Quilting Bee for Women 1:30 Crafts for Men 2:30 Book Cart on the Wards	9:30 AM Rhythm Band 2:00 Volunteers Reading, Visiting, Letter Writing 6:30 Learn Square and Round Dances with Your Friends

OR

Monday	Tuesday	Wednesday	Thursday	Friday
10 AM Informal Activities (Pool, Cards, Books, Checkers, Magazines) 1:30 Bowling Tournament 2:30 Coordinating Committee Meets (Plans for the Week)	10 AM Checker Tournament 1:30 Song Fest (Come and Sing with Your Friends) 2:30 Crafts (Join Your Friends in Making Something Useful)	10 AM Books and Magazines for Bed Patients 2:30 Rummage Sale (by Residents and for Residents in the Home) 6:00 PM Volunteers' Movies or Slides	10 AM Crafts for Men (Something for Someone Else) 1:30 Crafts for Women (Something for Someone Else) 2:30 Volunteers Visiting Bed Patients	10 AM Rag Rug Class 1:30 Bible Class 2:30 Skill – Ball Tourney

TABLE IV – continued

OR

10 AM Sheephead Tournament	10 AM Sewing Class	10 AM Copper Enameling, Ceramics	10 AM Rug Braiding Coffee Klatsch	10 AM Volunteers Reading, Visiting, Letter Writing
1:30 Birthday-Bingo Party	1:30 Dice Game Party	1:30 Residents- Participation Party	1:30 Informal Lounge Activities	1:30 Manicures, Shampoo, Charm Class (Women)
2:30 Folding Bandages for Community Chest	2:30 Shuffleboard	2:30 Book Review Club	2:30 News Discussion Group	2:30 Bumper Pool (Men)

OR

9:30 AM Decorating the Dining Room	9:30 AM Pitch-a-Penny	9:30 AM Making Scrapbooks for Orphanages	9:30 AM Men's Crafts	9:30 AM Chat and Chew – Coffee, Residents' Planning Committee
1:30 Get-Acquainted Club	1:30-4:00 Hobby Lobby – Open House and Craft Sale	1:30 Rummy Tournament	1:30 Crafts – Seed Pictures, Clove Apple Sachets	1:30 Popcorn Party
2:30 Ward Visits		2:30 Senior Citizens Club – with the Group from Town as Guests	6:30 Teenagers Night (Visiting, Games)	2:30 Quiet Games for Inactive People

TABLE IV – continued next page

TABLE IV – continued

OR

Monday	Tuesday	Wednesday	Thursdays	Friday
10 AM "I Remember" Hour (Let's Talk About It – Old Fashioned Kitchens, the Old School House, Life on the Farm) 1:30 Residents' Government Council – Steering Committee for the Home Program 2:30 Ward Visits	10 AM Women's Crafts – Knitting, Crocheting, Tatting, Embroidery– Get Your Supplies, Chat Together 1:30 Record Request Hour 2:30 Making Terraria –(Bedside Gardens for Bed Patients)	10 AM Camera Club (Have Your Picture Taken at Cost) 1:30 Cribbage Tournament 2:30 Reading Club – Read Aloud or Be Read to	10 AM Men's Carpentry Class 1:30 Help Your Neighbor Party (Cards and Dice) 2:30 Wheelchair Square Dance	10 AM Music Appreciation 1:30 Cootie Party 2:30 Reading, Writing Letters, Visiting on the Wards 6:30 Stage Club (With a Service Group from Town)

OR

Monday	Tuesday	Wednesday	Thursdays	Friday
10 AM Sing Rounds and Old Favorites 1:30 Dart Games 2:30 Surprise Party (Planned by Residents' Committee)	10 AM Good Fellowship Club (Write a Letter for a Friend, Read, Visit, Do an Errand for Another Resident) 1:30 Crafts – Popsicle Sticks – Salt Clay 6:30 Golden Agers (Guests from Town)	10 AM Cancer Pads for Community Chest 1:30 Home Government Meeting (Residents Program Planning) 2:30 Distributing Magazines – Books on Wards	10 AM Cards–Casino, Canasta, Pinochle, Parcheesi, Euchre 1:30 Coverall Party (Dice) 2:30 Decorating Committee – Bulletin Boards, Dining Room Tables Recreation	10 AM Woodenware Club – Breadboards, Whatnots Letter Holders, Boxes, Trays 1:30 Happy Hours Club (Residents Are Guests of the Town Club)

TABLE IV – continued

OR

Monday	Tuesday	Wednesday	Thursday	Friday
9:30 AM House Committee (Planning) / 1:30 Quoits / 2:30 Sing Along with Mitch	9:30 AM Visiting Committee (Residents Adopt New Admissions) / 1:30 Weaving Classes – Coffee Klatsch / 6:30 Weekly Movies	9:30 AM Arts and Crafts (Men and Women) / 1:30 Remotivation Class (Talkathon) / 2:30 Make a Corsage for Bed Patients	9:30 AM Bingo for Bed Patients / 1:30 Craft Sale Open House / 6:30 Bunco Party	9:30 AM Welcome Ladies – We Will Make Teaching Aids to be used by Retarded Children / 1:30 Poetry Reading / 2:30 Leather Crafts (Men and Women)

OR

Monday	Tuesday	Wednesday	Thursday	Friday
10 AM Chinese Checkers Tournament / 1:30 Home Membership Meeting / 2:30 Charm Class – Grooming (Women)	10 AM Bird Watchers Study Club / 1:30 Projects for Children in Hospital Pediatric Wards / 2:30 Card Tournament	10 AM Women's League of Voters Study Club / 1:30 Cooking Class / 6:30 Home Talent Show and Hymn Sing	10 AM Mending Party (Sewing Name Tags, Repairs, Sewing on Buttons for the Home) / 1:30 Rubber Horseshoes Tournament / 2:30 Jewelry Making Class	10 AM Beanbags / 1:30 Residents' Council Committee / 2:30 Library Circle Book – Cart on Wards

OR

Monday	Tuesday	Wednesday	Thursday	Friday
10 AM Shopping for Bed Patients / 1:30 Inner Circle (Residents' Program Planning) / 2:30 Mosaic Tile Class	10 AM Civics Class / 1:30 Horseracing / 2:30 Making Dolls for Underprivileged Children	10 AM Books Club / 1:30 Singo – Name the Tune / 6:30 Smoker – Cards and Smokes with Volunteers (Stag)	10 AM Chuck-a-Luck (Dice) / 1:30 Sewing Suzies / 2:30 Tea Time – (Conversation and Guessing Contests)	10 AM Conservation Club (Men) / 1:30 Service Club (Folding Napkins, Stuffing Envelopes, Counting Brochures) / 2:30 Travel Club (Guessing Contests, Guests, Slides and Movies, Talks)

perhaps the number of residents reached for the first time or any other simple statistics he might use. Reports of this sort also help volunteer goals, either showing what has been accomplished or what needs to be accomplished.

In some Homes, "Report A" (a form for which follows) lists the names of all residents in the Home with dates at the top of the page; goals set for reaching everyone are often more nearly reached by residents and volunteers being aware of the records lying on the table in the craft room; the resident looks up the patient, for instance, to whom he can read the newspaper, for whom to write a letter, urge the withdrawn resident with no activity check after his name to come down to the card tournament or play a bedside game.

Simple checks should take only a few minutes of time daily if done immediately following an activity; some Homes instead of using a check, put a simple code letter in the space indicating what the activity was: S (singalong), C (craft), G (game), M (movies), V (visiting), R (rides), etc. An able resident can take roll call on the report sheet which saves time for the activity aide, who perhaps prefers not to report large groups like movies, bingo or birthday party attendance; often he can remember who was there if the group isn't too large. Keeping a large posted sheet of residents' names with gold stars has spurred attendance and kept an easy record.

Reports B and C are examples of other types of check sheets which are used. Each Home can design its own form based on its own program.

TABLE V

REPORT A

ACTIVITY RECORDS FOR INDIVIDUAL RESIDENTS

Working Days of the Month	Apr 1	2	5	6	7	8	9	12	13	14	15	16	19	20	21	22	23	26	27	28	29
Names of Residents																					

TABLE VI
REPORT B

MONTHLY PARTICIPATION RECORD

(to be filled out by person in charge of the activity)

	1	2	3	4	5	6	7	8	9	10	11	12	13	14	15	16	17	18	19	20	21	22	23	24	25	26	27	28	29	30	31	TOTAL
Visits By Prog. Dir.																																
Vol. Visits																																
Letter Writing For																																
Reading To																																
Library																																
Church Services																																
Special Events																																
Parties																																
Entertainment																																
Birthdays – Ind.																																
Records – Phono.																																
Music																																
Movies																																
Small Games																																
Bingo																																
Bowling																																
Arts																																
Ceramics																																
Chenille & Beads																																
Knitting & Sewing																																
Leather																																
Mosaic Tile																																
Weaving																																
Newspaper – Hosp.																																
Volunteers																																

TABLE VII
REPORT C

A report on therapeutic attempts in a broad program might be useful to other activity personnel interested in the same goals, making studies and using joint referrals.

THERAPIST REPORT

(Showing number of residents reached daily as well as the type of activity)

Therapist .... *Week of* ....

Type of Activity	Monday	Tuesday	Wednesday	Thursday	Friday
Passive Therapy					
Individual Therapy					
Music Therapy					
Industrial Therapy					
Daily Workers					
Arts and Crafts					
Movies (daytime)					
Drama					
Square Dancing					
Games					
Community Singing					
Remotivation					
Evening Program					

TABLE VIII

REPORT D

Budget Report

(To be filled out by the activity aide and submitted to the superintendent or his superior at the end of the year, or the end of the month, or to be used as an anticipated budget.)

Craft Supplies ....

Art Supplies ....

Games ....

Movies ....

Refreshments ....

Prizes and Presents ....

Decorations ....

Major Equipment ....

Office Supplies and Equipment ....

Miscellaneous ....

Total ....

Sales of Patients' Craft Items ....

Total ....

Chapter VI

EVALUATION

Accentuate the positive

RESIDENTS' PROGRESS RECORD IN ACTIVITIES

A CARD FILE for residents' names, ages, religion, physical handicaps, special interests and favorite foods, with room for additional comments on hobbies can be added as the program progresses.

An infirmary registrar fills in the admission sheets with hobbies of those residents being admitted; proper referrals are then given to the activity aide and the volunteers.

Doctors, nurses or nearest of kin may be interested in an activity report, an area in which they do not always see the resident showing coordination, muscular control or use of his arms and hands, for instance; his reactions and his improvements may come as a surprise to others responsible for him, or perhaps they feel he should be accomplishing more in the activity program.

Report E

Evaluation in a Narrative Report

A narrative annual report often tells a great deal that numbers and statistics fail to do; describing a program concisely, summarizing accomplishments and perhaps needs, may speak more eloquently of what's happening than pages of figures.

This report is submitted to the administrator at the end of the calendar year by the leader, in this case, the occupational therapist; the administrator may want to submit it to the newspaper for publicity or refer it to his trustees.

Activity Annual Report

The activity program at the Infirmary was resumed on March 25, 1965. For the first two months, the schedule consisted mainly of ward contacts and shop activities daily and bingo once weekly. With the arrival of warmer weather, outdoor activities including horseshoes, croquet, and shuffleboard were added to the program.

In June, an occupational therapy assistant was added to the staff. Subsequently, the program broadened further to include weekly bunco games and card parties held in the dining room. More residents were also brought to the craft shop for cards, bunco and crafts during the open shop hours.

When cooler fall weather puts a stop to outdoor activities, dartball and bowling were tried indoors. Response was quite favorable, so teams were formed and a bowling tournament was set up, batting average being kept for dartball. These activities will continue into April, when prizes will be awarded.

The last week of September saw the issuing of a newsletter, the **Infirmary News,** put out by the occupational therapy department, and consists of reports of current activities as well as poems, jokes, puzzles, etc., contributed by the residents. Response has been quite favorable, residents looking forward to each new issue with several regular contributors.

During November, another new activity, the Investor's Club, was started, with thirty-five residents participating. Each member receives the same amount of imaginary money to "invest." Records are kept of the stock he buys and dividends he would receive, and at the end of six months the players whose "investments" are worth the most will receive prizes.

Special events during the year included a July 4th outing in the grove, the annual picnic, several ball games, a bus trip, three trips to the new zoo, a Halloween party and dance and a Christmas carol sing.

The three rooms which comprise the department have been well-used. During the open shop hours, the double room is often filled to overflowing. The single room is used largely for storage and preparation of craft materials and is not always suitable for craft activities or card games since the residents who do painting prefer a little more quiet.

The OTR and OTA attended the Southwestern District County Home Activity Institute at Honwell, Wisconsin, on

October 16th, and the Wisconsin Recreation Association meeting at the Coach House, Houghton, on November 6th. Craft sales were held on August 24th and 25th, and on December 14th. Sales totaled $100.25 and $113.45.

Attendance statistics for the year are as follows:

Month	Recreation	Ward and Shop	Totals
March	—	53	53
April	302	426	728
May	386	416	802
June	533	371	908
July	685	391	1076
August	671	471	1142
September	909	582	1491
October	875	664	1539
November	865	614	1479
December	925	671	1626
Year Totals	6151	4726	10,877

...., OTR

TABLE IX

RECORD F

RESIDENT'S PROGRESS RECORD IN ACTIVITIES

Name of Resident ....

Age: .... Birthday ....

Physical Condition:

Ambulatory .... Hearing .... Coordination   — Good

Semi   Poor

    Ambulatory   Visual handicaps .... Muscular control — Good

Bedfast .... Use of arms and hands .... Mental condition — Good

---

Activities:

Occupation:

Hobbies:

Interests:

Social:

Church:

Club or lodge affiliation:

Dates Introduced to Activities:

Dates:

                                             Activities:

Comments on Reaction:

                                             Attitude: Nonreceptive

                                                       Receptive

                                             Interest: Good

                                                   Indifferent

General Benefits and Improvements:

                         ....

                                     Signed by professional worker

TABLE X
RECORD G

RESIDENT RESPONSE TO TYPE OF ACTIVITY (MEDICAL REFERRAL)

Individual

Activity Therapy Department **Resident Progress Report**

(Working Closely with the Nurse or Doctor)

Name **Birth Date** **Religion**

Medical Status: **Restrictions:**

Ventrical hernia, slight hearing None. Limits self when
defect, A. S. necessary.

Remarks:

Was seclusive and depressed before activity program. Now cheerful, a leader and excellent help with handicapped residents teaching them to play. Calm, and thoughtful of others. Completely accepted by all.

Date	Type of Activity	Response	Date Changes
12/1/64	Outdoor	Plays well and stimulates others to join.	1/1/64 None Remains Consistent
	Cards	Plays intelligently, eagerly and happily.	
	Table games	Plays cheerfully to be of help to others.	
11/1/65	Crafts	Does whatever she can to help with limited eyesight.	
	Parties	Always joins and enjoys self, even dances occasionally.	

EVALUATING THE RESIDENT

It is necessary to know the resident as well as possible — attendants on the wards giving baths and working closely with him are often helpful.

1. Does the resident have a chance to take part in planning specific activities in the Home?

2. Are the resident's needs studied carefully and adapted to the program?

3. Can the resident evaluate the program through questionnaires, a resident council or other specific requests on what he'd like in a program?

4. Are individual special interests, talents, physical abilities, sex, religious, and cultural backgrounds considered?

5. Is there a chance for the resident to see improvement, accomplishment and success in a program planned to help him achieve as much as he's able?

6. Does encouragement, recognition and approval go with his taking part?

7. Does the program give him a sense of belonging and having some importance in the Home?

8. Is the resident learning new interests and developing helpful skills?

9. Is resident helped to develop and learn through new activities?

10. Is effort made to determine improved change in his attitude, behavior, social and physical?

EVALUATING THE LEADER

1. Does the activity staff closely cooperate in working with the rest of the Home personnel, attending daily staff meetings, informing them of the program and receiving individual referrals of residents with whom to work?

2. Are the leader's responsibilities related to his training?

3. Does the leader have a chance to develop skills by attending schools or institutes, workshops and professional meetings?

4. Do the leaders at every level have supervision and direction?

5. Is every resource — equipment and man power — in the Home utilized to expand the program?

6. Does each leader have his duties as well as the goals of the program stated in writing?

7. Does the leader give thought to the future in budgets, facilities and equipment as well as program?

8. Does budget planning correspond with the achievements to be reached in the program, a budget which contributes directly to the needs of the program?

9. Is equipment adequate and are areas attractive?

10. Are reports and records kept for permanent use in the Home?

11. Is there good communication among activity staff members and among other departments?

12. Can the leader evoke good response with his staff, directing and inspiring them rather than dictating?

13. Does the leader keep in mind definite needs and individual differences among residents?

EVALUATING THE PROGRAM

1. Do activities offer the greatest active participation by the greatest number of residents?

2. Are activities centered around a stated goal for the program?

3. Is there a balance of social and physical activities, crafts, games?

4. Is there appropriate balance between individual and group activities?

5. Do activities provide for the resident making some contribution to the community, in some way taking part in community life?

6. Is the program judged only by the number of participants or by their interest, enthusiasm and satisfaction?

7. Are activities judged not only on their number and variety but also on their effectiveness?

8. Does the program teach skills and offer materials for continued activity during evenings and weekends?

9. Does programming allow for working with individuals?

10. Do all activities agree with the nursing goals of the Home?

11. Is the program broad enough to provide for a wide range of interests for individuals?

12. Does the program change as the needs of the residents change?

13. Does the program kindle group consciousness and residents' responsibility to one another?

14. Can the program scheduled be continued over a length of time?

Chapter VII

VOLUNTEERS

We should be less willing to assist and do for, but more willing to encourage self help and teach how.

RECRUITMENT

SPEAKING TO JUST the right community leader, a relative or friend of one of the residents may trigger the start in a program; later, as the program grows, larger numbers of volunteers may be encouraged as the Home finds assignments for them. But often enthusiasm in recruitment leads to large numbers of potential volunteers being given orientation, only to discover five of them can't be kept busy watering the flowers or delivering the mail all afternoon. Two or three assignments of standing around finishes them off, probably never to return. A request for the number of volunteers needed, then, is important; but if the activity aide needs five volunteers to work with her Tuesday afternoons from 1 PM to 3:30 PM she ought to ask for eight and train them, since there are usually dropouts among volunteers because of transportation problems, obligations to their families and other circumstances beyond their control which may arise.

No matter how small the community or how isolated it is, there are evidences of success stories in volunteer recruitment. Sometimes the chairman of the group is also the chauffeur, and is responsible for bringing five people for the day or for the afternoon to the Home. Volunteers must sign up for certain days and get a substitute if they are unable to come.

In screening recruits, one Home asks volunteers to submit applications and a "recommendation written by someone else," sent to the chairman of their volunteer group. Screening sometimes presents problems, but volunteers should understand that their assignment in the Home is on a trial basis, to their advantage as well as the advantage to the Home.

Usually the best recruitment is done by the volunteers themselves, who know their friends and neighbors well enough to
decide if they would qualify in this work. Also a good volunteer's
enthusiasm for her work, if sincere, is contagious, and other
volunteers will be anxious to follow the Pied Piper.

A local architect loaned out models of the new nursing home,
complete with blueprints, floor plans and drawings to publicize
the Home program of recruitment. A small, interested group
of volunteers was expanded by each valuable volunteer bringing
a friend to recruitment meetings. Form letters sent to county
wide church groups or organizations listed by the Chamber of
Commerce have often brought in volunteers.

Many times, interested groups sponsoring monthly parties have
been broken down to individuals who come more often after
receiving in-service training and work in some specialized assignment set up on a regular basis in the Home, giving more hours.

Most Homes and hospitals have found it advisable to announce
to prospective volunteers that the first ten hours of hospital work
are a probation period. At the end of this period, the hospital
notifies the volunteer organization on the aptitude of its volunteers.
Recommendations are made for permanent assignment of the volunteer to the department in which she served, her transfer to
another department where she would be more suited, or with-
drawal of the volunteer not adapted for this work. The community organization then notifies each of the volunteers and tries
to find another field of service for them.

Home personnel encourage community club meetings being
brought into the Homes on a regular basis — local card or chess
or checker clubs, for instance.

Auxiliary members bring articles from many countries to display in the reception room, each volunteer explaining the item
and its history.

Residents bring antiques from their rooms for a similar display.

Form Letters Used in Recruitment

Dear Students at Toltseville University:

*We are asking your help in bringing a volunteer program
to the aged and infirm at Trent County Home. With over*

eighty-eight residents, we have a limited staff, limited space, and limited time to help these people. Many people have had no visitors for months or years. Many of them are too shy, lacking initiative to enter into activity programs. They need individual attention in being urged into a new interest. The very fact that a volunteer is willing to take the time and make the effort to come to the Home without being paid for this service, but is still interested enough to help, has a happy effect on them.

We think your group would like a part in this modern approach to the large and challenging problem of the loneliness of old age. We need willing, dependable, cheerful volunteers. It's you and what you can give of yourself in time and friendship that would be helpful in this program.

And we can promise you great rewards: the deep gratitude of these people, the good will toward the community here and a personal pride and satisfaction for you.

The residents at the Trent County Home have a volunteer group which sometimes take them for rides, and on alternate Wednesdays, come as beauticians working with women residents; a religious leader visiting the Home makes tapes of their singing which she plays back to them on her next visit.

We would prefer to have volunteer groups come in afternoons; but if this isn't possible, we would like you from 6 PM to 7:30 PM, since these people retire early. We are especially anxious for reliable groups who will be here on time and who won't let us down — it's a very hard thing to face residents who have been sitting waiting an hour for a volunteer group which has never called to cancel their schedule. Escorting wheelchairs down to the recreation room also takes a great deal of employees' time; part of the enjoyment of any activity is their getting ready for it — putting on a clean shirt for the company, assured that "you'll be there because you said you would."

We will appreciate hearing from you.

MRS. DELVIN RELTE, *Assistant Supt.*
Trent County Home
Dancaster, Wisconsin

Dear Students at Toltseville University

We have drawn up activities the Toltseville University students might bring as volunteers.

The art department: working with the residents making decorations, trimming Christmas trees, tables, and rooms for the holidays, displaying an art exhibit, sketching residents or teaching sketching to a small group of residents.

A dramatic club: giving a plays dress rehearsal at the Home; a debate team practice; doing pantomining, charades, or guessing games with residents; playing bingo or holding game nights, the Home furnishing the prizes and refreshments so there would be no expense involved.

The music department: encouraging singing or directing a resident rhythm band.

Phys ed department: folk dancing or square dancing exhibitions.

Library or literary groups: discussion classes, reading club, or literary club.

All of our residents need your friendship. Will you adopt a floor to entertain or visit regularly, perhaps one night every week or every alternate week?

You will find these oldsters anxious to please, and to be pleasant, and anxious to be accepted by you. You will find them unusually responsive and appreciative. They will like you and will be anxious for you to like them.

I will be glad to come to your group to discuss this project, perhaps show a short film on county homes, display simple crafts made by residents in our county home, or hold workshops with you and the residents learning simple games or taking part in beanbag, ringtoss, bowling, or horseshoe tournaments. I am available any afternoon or evening. Contact may be made directly with me by sending a card, giving the date and time of your next meeting or, if you prefer to call the Home, ask for me, and arrange to schedule a date and time.

Sincerely,

Mrs. Delvin Relte, *Assistant Supt.*
Trent County Home
Dancaster, Wisconsin

Releases for Newspapers and Radio, in Recruiting Volunteers

We are proud of our .... Home, dedicated to the care of oldsters. The staff there works with residents who have varied and numerous needs and who would be helped in knowing that you are interested in them. Can your hobby group meet with these people once a week? You will find real pride and satisfaction in this work and a better understanding of the aged. Such hobbies as sewing, checkers, cooking, cards, music and books — would work in nicely with our program. Call . . .

* * * * * *

Old people express both pleasure and happy surprise that unpaid people come as volunteers to ease their lives and help them to a happier outlook. They need your social club or church group to help with card parties, smokers, checker tournaments, hobby groups or news discussion classes. Many residents have had few or no visitors for months or years. They feel forgotten and isolated. Will you help restore their faith in you and confidence in themselves?

* * * * * *

Would you like to be granddaughter or grandson to an oldster? Give him the encouragement he needs with a ward card party, a birthday party, or a monthly entertainment. This isn't an appeal for money but for your time and service, something much more valuable, something only you can give. Arrange for a worker from .... Home to come and talk to your club or church group and explain the needs of the residents. Call . . . .

* * * * * *

Everyone knows that time goes faster if you have something to do. Home residents are often hospitalized for lengthy

stays. Ill, lonely, and away from home,
they need encouragement. Can your club
help by giving an hour a month for a
birthday party on a ward, an informal
sewing class, a ward fudge party, or a
card game? Call ....

Orientation in Visitation

If the volunteer comes to visit a resident she hasn't met, she
ought to check first with the activity aide for a resident who
needs visitors and she should be told something about each resident — where did he live, what work or hobbies has he had, who
were his friends, how does he keep himself busy and useful in
the Home, in what does he seem interested and what are his
physical limitations? She must also get permission to bring him
food, take him outside or for a ride, or shop for him.

An activity aide gives to volunteers going to the wards baskets
with games and apples for prizes, assigns them numbers of rooms
and names of residents; each volunteer visits four rooms in an
afternoon. Volunteers are given a paper, pad and pencil to jot
down "helps," program ideas or new activities which the Home
might launch. The activity aide also lists helps in starting a conversation which they find handy and useful. In turn, the volunteers note residents who never have visitors, an item of great
value to an activity aide who attempts to keep in close touch
with over 200 residents.

One Home has made up cards for volunteers' use giving the
resident's name and notes which would help a visitor: "Deaf,"
"Likes to visit," "Loves to read," "Likes to do her own reading
and writes beautifully," "LaFarge (a nearby village) area," "Very
hard to understand," "Likes attention," "Quite confused," "Likes
to crochet," "Loves seed catalogues," "He is blind," "Methodist,"
"Westby area," "Sons are missionaries," "Deaf-mute," "Ill—unable
to visit," "Uses feet in place of hands."

On meeting the resident, she shakes hands, but lets him do
the squeezing — an arthritic may be hurt by too firm a grip; she
may greet him instead with a gentle touch or a pat on the arm,
perhaps making a leading statement about some of his interests,
without asking "How are you?" commenting cheerfully on some-

thing he is wearing, using, or something in the room.

Never apologetic about her visit, she comes with the feeling that the resident is eager for personal contact. The resident who seems to reject the visitor may be the one who is most anxious for friendship but doesn't know how to accept it. The volunteer may make several visits before both of them find conversation in how the resident feels; if the conversation cannot be broken off after fifteen minutes or more, the volunteer may excuse herself by saying she has other residents she must visit. Her smile and personal contact are the finest gifts she can bring.

Selecting a place where the resident can see her without eye strain or looking into the light, she should avoid such subjects as gossip, making comparisons with illness of others or commenting on the way the doctor is caring for the resident.

The visitor's relationship to the resident is as a friend and companion, performing friendly little services, helping him realize there is someone who cares for him and is interested in him.

She is a good listener to the lonely resident who needs someone to talk to and in whom he can confide; conversation may indicate ways of activating him in latent interests and talents, but anything which seems to be a problem should be referred to the activity aide. The visitor, aware of the resident's concern, does not contradict, but lets him talk about things that interest him, being considerate of his feelings. On each visit she gets him to do something, commenting on his progress if it's good, treating him as an adult and an equal, never "talking down" to him in a patronizing way. She may be able to direct his past experiences toward developing a new life in the nursing home, visiting him as often as possible, and telephoning him between visits if the Home approves.

In the event of personal conflict in her relationship with the resident and if the visitor cannot completely accept him, she ought to ask to visit another resident next time. In the interests of friendship, she may remember him on special days or occasionally bring some small surprise approved by the Home.

It is not for the volunteer to judge residents, not for her to be a social worker, pastor, medical doctor or lawyer. But it is important that she completely accept him, good or bad as his disposition may be, and correctly interpret his delusions as such, convincing as they may be.

Services which can also be performed by the "Friendly Visitor" (another name for "volunteer") might be to encourage him to attend activities; to listen to certain radio or TV programs; develop new hobbies and reawaken old ones; help find outlets for his handicrafts; read to him and write letters for him; play games with him, and with permission from the nurse, do his shopping; take him for a ride or to visit some old friend; help him down the hall with wheelchair or walker; bring a project from the community or church with which he can help, or find something which gives him special recognition in which he can be complimented.

There are always a number of residents so physically handicapped that they can't be reached in more active ways; but a dependable, willing, cheerful Friendly Visitor can be a great morale booster. A short visit radiating hope and good will for a lonely resident can make life worthwhile from one visit to the next.

Workshops

The most common expression of helplessness among new volunteer-recruits is, "I always wanted to help, but I never knew what I could do!" A workshop is an attempt to teach volunteers some simple skills which might help in making friendships, easy ways of bringing people together happily, reaching the lonely and depressed, the inactive and withdrawn. A day or two should be given to a workshop, perhaps one day for crafts and another day for games.

Working in the area where volunteers will later be assigned and working with residents is important; part of the benefit of the workshop is the assignment-situation — learning that residents work slowly, often don't hear or see well, can't easily learn new games unless they are simple, and shouldn't be bothered with complicated rules — that they don't have the strength in their hands to do all crafts. Other observations should be made in this first experience.

GAME WORKSHOP. Perhaps each volunteer could bring a

favorite game the resident knows and a deck of cards to each table of residents. Most old people like "66," casino, crazy eights, pinochle, Chinese checkers, caroms, sheepshead, double solitaire, old maid and a variety of other card games as well as quizzes, riddles, icebreakers or puzzles. Volunteers can serve as game instructors at tables set-up and numbered; after fifteen to twenty minutes of playing, the volunteer rotates, taking the game to the next table, teaching it, and continuing to all tables. Prizes should never be the only motivation in playing a game; however, a drawing, favors, or passing a small treat makes for sociability and a pleasant surprise. The aged and infirm ought not to be placed in the position of competition; games of chance are much more acceptable if they must learn games new to them. Prizes should come just as a special treat, not the sole incentive for activity.

CRAFT WORKSHOP. Activity aides have been enthusiastic about invitations to nearby summer institutes where a professional crafts person from national recreation association or other agency teaches low-cost creative crafts suitable for work with the aged and infirm. A $1.00 fee and each participant furnishing her own salvage material used in making four items make it possible for each aide to return to the Home with four samples to show residents, and the skill to teach residents.

At the craft workshop the volunteers may bring salvage materials with which to make an item. The finished craftwork is displayed at each table with patterns and materials ready to begin work on the craft; for the inexperienced, tile mosaics, macaroni crafts, or copper tooling are easy starts.

Other Home craft workshops have been conducted by each volunteer bringing a craft idea and the materials to work with a few residents and perhaps a few other volunteers. Or perhaps the activity aide sets up the materials for the residents, volunteers watching and assisting the resident when required but never taking over the production. Even if the volunteer thinks she can do it "better and faster," she must be reminded that "it's the patient, not the product" one hopes to develop in program goals. The resident must do all or as much of it as he can. Threading needles, keeping supplies ready, wiping up spills and showing the resident how, through encouragement, are valuable volunteer contributions.

Another type of game workshop would be in teaching a few new games to volunteers along with the residents in the same fashion but spending fifteen minutes teaching coverall, for instance, to the group of volunteers, who then disperse one at each table to teach the game to the oldsters. The activity aide starts a new game at the first table which can be shown in a few minutes, actually playing the game, starting by throwing the dice and putting on the markers, explaining the rules as they play, making it easy. As the game progresses, of course, he moves to the next tables, teaching residents and volunteers at each table. If there are six tables, he may need a volunteer who knows the games — bunco, keeno, and card bingo, one at a time down the line at each table. Later, mimeographed rules of the games may be distributed to the volunteers as referrals when they visit the Home and invite a resident to play.

ORGANIZING VOLUNTEERS

Groups

OCCASIONAL ENTERTAINMENT GROUPS (spectator types of activity). These groups come occasionally during the year though not on a regular basis. It is taken for granted that most nursing homes have a variety of entertainment brought into the Home by groups of volunteers usually welcome if the date, time and type of entertainment are approved by the superintendent or someone representing him, such as the activity aide. An understanding must be reached, however, as to the number of entertainers, the size of the room available, whether or not a microphone, movie projector, or screen are necessary, as well as suitable areas, such as a dark room for an afternoon movie. If it's an outdoor activity, some alternate program or area must be available in case of bad weather or any other unpredicted emergency.

Complaints are made in all nursing homes about volunteer groups who fail to show up once they have been announced; the Home is ready and often has taken a great deal of time preparing residents, escorting them to the chapel or recreation hall only to be disappointed by volunteers never arriving. The activity aide should always be prepared with games, movie, music, or a party packet to avert such a tragedy, and the volunteer chairman should be contacted as soon as possible to iron out the misunderstanding and to discover how to prevent this from reoccurring. Better yet, the aide should call the chairman responsible before the activity is announced to check once again on the date, time and place.

The activity aide or the person responsible in the Home should be at the door to greet the group on arrival, direct them to facilities for wraps and other conveniences, stay with them throughout the activity, and until each volunteer has left, thanking them, of course, and if the program warrants it, asking them to name a date for a return program.

Volunteers' programs have included movies and slides, children's performances, religious services, favorite old-time hymn sings, kitchen bands, teenage baton "twirlers," tap dancing, choir, pantomime, folk singing, combos or orchestras, toe dancing, flannel talks, a high school class play rehearsal, debate team workout, style show, music recitals, etc.

GROUPS SPONSORING MONTHLY SOCIAL PARTIES. Sometimes the volunteer groups sponsor monthly social parties working with large groups of residents with bingo, bunco or birthday parties continuing in the summer with picnics or outdoor events for residents. Groups like the Junior League, Federated Women's Clubs, and church or business organizations have proven valuable, often providing and serving some simple refreshments, bringing the entertainment, simple prizes, birthday gifts, "live" music, or another activity. One sponsoring group sends out individual invitations to the residents having birthdays that month though all the residents are invited; each celebrating resident receives an individual cake.

Volunteers are trained to help escort the residents to these activity areas and back again afterward, whether outside or in the recreation or dining room, since often the many wheelchair residents require so much help the affair could never be conducted without this assistance. Birthday celebrations become important if the celebrants are seated in a special place — a stage

or in front of the fireplace — given paper hats and seated facing
the lighted cake.

Men's service organizations like Lions, Kiwanis or Rotary, or
again, church groups, have conducted stag parties for men only,
playing a group game like bingo or a simple dice game, passing
out "smokes", a cold drink or fruit, refreshments always being
approved by the nurse beforehand.

"Smokers" seem an acceptable way of reaching many men
residents; each volunteer sits at a separate card table and attracts
players to his table for a favorite game. Men volunteers usually
can be scheduled for early evening activities arriving at 6:30 PM
and staying for an hour, and still be home by 8 PM for any
evening obligation with their families.

VOLUNTEERS WORKING REGULARLY WITH SMALL SPECIAL INTER-
EST GROUPS. These groups work with individual residents or small
groups of residents in some special interest, game, craft or hobby.

A county home chaplain contacting his County Council of
Churches — 450 members who were organized in twenty-one
church circles in the county — suggested that they organize a
daily volunteer program in the Home; each of the twenty-one
circles, with five to eight members in each circle, come one afternoon a month, so that residents now have a program five days a
week from 1 PM to 3 PM. The activity aide talked to several
church circles describing her work and the assistance needed from
volunteers, previous to their signing up for a special day each
month. Two days of workshops with volunteers were held in the
Home, training volunteers in individual skills with games and
crafts.

The aide meets with the chairman of the groups the third Tuesday of each month and on a large calendar for the following
month draws up activities, listing the telephone number of the
chairman for each day and naming the activity planned and the
responsibilities which the Home has for the activity, such as
providing refreshments, supplying paste and paper for crafts,
music, furnishing the games, etc.; discussing together in what
room the activity will be held; how many residents will be
reached, etc. If this is carefully done, no further volunteer contacts have to be made, the volunteer chairman and activity aide

each having a copy of the calendar.

The program in this instance includes: Mondays, crafts; Tuesdays, games; Wednesdays, Bible Class; Thursdays, hair care; Fridays, "fellowship": slides, community sings, parties or entertainment from the outside.

Community groups such as Senior Citizens, Golden Agers, or church groups meet regularly in the Homes, holding meetings to which residents are invited, satisfying the need for "belonging." Pen pals and Bible classes make for happy oldsters. Women's auxiliaries have dependably provided valuable and ambitious projects for raising money for "extras" for the Home or sponsoring weekly special interest groups, games, crafts or hobbies.

TABLE XI

VOLUNTEER ENTERTAINMENT PROGRAM RECORD

.... Home

Date .... 196.......

Name of Group or Individual ....

Contact Person ....

Address ....

Telephone ....

Time Expected and Date .... 196.......

Place ....

Transportation ....

Program ....

....

....

Refreshments Provided by Group ....

Refreshments Provided by Home ....

Equipment Provided by Group ....

Equipment Provided by Home ....

Resident Attendance ....

Evaluation by Worker ....

....

....

....

....

Thank You Letter Written by ....

Mechanics of Organization

The Home Auxiliary

Home auxiliaries are often organized either as a service group assigned to work in the Home, raise money for equipment or supplies for the Home, or both. In a county with a total population of only twenty thousand people, the auxiliary has realized one thousand paid auxiliary memberships in door-to-door canvassing; in fact, the auxiliary was organized through the leadership of a county welfare worker prior to the construction of the building of the Home.

Each year this volunteer group has given $1,000.00 in gifts to the Home. Among the members one hundred and twenty have "adopted" residents. Since there are only fifty-five residents in the Home, each resident has two volunteers assigned to assist him in personal services, take him for rides, remember him on holidays and his birthday, and visit with him frequently.

A nurse-supervisor prevented ill feeling that might be shown by employees when the auxiliary made its first visit to the Home, by successfully urging 90 per cent of the employees to join the auxiliary, attend meetings, vote, and develop good volunteer-employee relations; employees here strengthen the auxiliary and Home relationships by working as auxiliary members.

Constitution and By-laws

Suggested by Constitution and By-Laws Committee:

> Evelyn ...., Chairman
> Eileen ....
> Evelyn ....
> Marjorie ....

Article I: Name and Purpose

Section 1. The name of this organization shall be Jameson County Home and Hospital Auxiliary.

Section 2. The purpose of this organization shall be to promote the welfare of the Jameson County Home and Hospital through ways approved by the board of trustees.

Wolf, Stephanie R

ID:39314100132117
617.482044 Sp462 1994
Spinal cord injury :
\Yarkony, Gary M.
date:4/18/2001,17:45
paid: .10
 billed: $.10
change:

type:CASH
Paid in full

This purpose shall be accomplished by interpretation of the hospital to the public, through the service to the hospital and its patients, and through fund raising in a manner satisfactory to the board of trustees and in harmony with the planning of the community.

Article II: Membership

Section 1. Membership in the auxiliary shall be open to all persons who are interested in the Jameson County Home and Hospital.

Section 2. There shall be the following types of members:

A. Active members who shall pay annual dues of $1.00 and who shall participate in active service programs of the auxiliary.

B. Associate members who shall pay annual dues of $1.00 and who shall be interested in the purposes of the auxiliary but who do not participate actively.

C. Life members who shall pay $25.00. A life member shall be exempt from further payment of dues.

D. All hospital volunteers must be paid members.

Section 3. Any member in good standing shall have the right to vote, to participate in meetings, and to hold office in the auxiliary.

Article III: Board of Directors

Section 1. The board of directors shall consist of those who are: (a) officers of the auxiliary (b) six elected directors of the auxiliary (c) chairman of standing committees (d) the Home and hospital administrator and (e) one representative from the activities or occupational therapy department of the institution.

Section 2. Two directors shall be elected annually to serve three year terms, but shall not be eligible to serve more than two consecutive terms. The initial year two members shall be elected for one year, two members for two years, and two members for three years.

Section 3. Any vacancy occurring among the directors prior to an election shall be filled by the vote of the board of directors from candidates presented by the nominating committee. Such a director shall serve for the unexpired term of her predecessor.

Section 4. The board of directors shall meet alternate months the first year for purposes of education and expansion of membership. After the initial year quarterly meetings shall be held, one of these being the annual meeting. Special meetings of the directors may be called by the president for the transacting of business and must be called by her at the request of the board of directors or at the written request of any five members of the board. The time and place of such special meetings shall be determined by the president.

Section 5. Notice of all meetings of the board of directors, both regular and special, shall be given by the secretary.

Article IV: Officers

Section 1. The officers of the auxiliary shall be: A president, a vice president, a secretary, a treasurer, chairmen of of standing committees, and such assistants as may be necessary.

Section 2. Officers of the auxiliary shall serve for a term of two years. Officers shall not be eligible to serve more than two consecutive terms. This limitation shall not apply to the office of the treasurer.

Section 3. The initial year a president and vice president shall be elected for a two year term, to be elected thereafter in the even years, the vice president to succeed the president. The initial year a secretary and treasurer shall be elected for a one year term, to be elected thereafter in the odd years for a two year term.

Article V: Duties and Powers of Officers and Board

Section 1. The executive power of the auxiliary shall be vested in the board of directors who shall have charge of the affairs and funds of the auxiliary and shall have the power and authority to do and perform all acts and functions in accordance with these by-laws.

Section 2. The president shall be the chief executive officer of the auxiliary. She shall preside at all meetings of the auxiliary, board of directors, and executive committee. The president shall be an ex-officio member of all committees except the nominating committee. The president shall appoint the chairmen of all standing committees, subject to the approval of the board of directors. She shall read a report on the activities of the auxiliary annually to the board of trustees and to the auxiliary membership at its annual meeting.

Section 3. The treasurer shall be the chief fiscal officer of the auxiliary. She shall receive all funds paid to the auxiliary and shall deposit such funds in the name of the auxiliary in such banks as the executive committee may designate from time to time. She shall pay all bills for the auxiliary after these bills have been certified and approved for payment by the president and the chairman of the committee incurring the bill. She shall keep or cause to be kept in suitable form, detailed accounts of the assets, liabilities, receipts, and disbursements of the auxiliary. The books shall be open at all times for examination or audit by the auditors or such representatives of the executive committee as it may designate from time to time. She shall render an annual report to the auxiliary and to the board of trustees, and the books shall be audited annually. The treasurer shall be bonded in such amount and with such surety as the executive committee may determine. The expense of the bond shall be borne by the auxiliary.

Section 4. The secretary shall keep an accurate record of the proceedings of the meetings of the auxiliary, the board of directors, and the executive committed. The records shall be open at all times to reasonable inspection by any member of the auxiliary. She shall give notice of the meetings of the auxiliary, the board of directors, and executive committee.

Article VI: Executive Committee

Section 1. There shall be an executive committee whose membership shall consist of the officers of the auxiliary, the immediate past-president of the auxiliary, the administrator of the Home and hospital, and such chairman of standing committees as the president may designate with the approval of the board of directors.

Section 2. Standing committees shall be (a) Service (b) Membership (c) Entertainment (d) Publicity and (e) Awards and Recognition.

Section 3. The executive committee shall exercise all powers of the board of directors during the interim between meetings of the board of directors.

Section 4. All actions of the executive committee shall be subject to ratification by the board of directors of the hospital auxiliary.

Article VII: Committees

Section 1. There shall be such standing committees as are necessary for the conduct of the business and program of the auxiliary. The president shall appoint the chairman of each committee with the approval of the executive committee as soon as possible after the annual meeting of the auxiliary. The personnel of each committee shall consist of such members as may be designated by the chairman of the committee with the approval of the president.

Article VIII: Nominating Committee

Section 1. There shall be a nominating committee elected annually by the membership. It shall consist of five members. Two of these members shall be members of the board of directors, two shall be from the general membership and one shall be the chairman of the outgoing nominating committee. The committee shall elect its own chairman.

Section 2. The nominating committee shall prepare a slate of nominees for officers, board of directors, honorary members, and the incoming nominating committee.

Section 3. Nominations may be made from the floor. A majority vote of those present and voting is necessary in order to place these names on the ballot.

Section 4. The nominating committee shall function throughout the year to name candidates for any vacancies among the officers or board of directors, and to submit these names to the board of directors for election by the board to fill the unexpired terms.

Article IX: Meetings

Section 1. There shall be meetings alternate months the first year, quarterly meetings thereafter, one of the latter being the annual meeting.

Section 2. The time and place of meetings may be designated by the president and/or the executive committee. The publicity committee, with the secretary shall be responsible for notification to the membership.

Section 3. The annual meeting shall be held in May of each year for the election of officers and standing committees, and such other business as may properly come before the meeting.

Section 4. The president or the majority of the board of directors may call a special meeting of the general membership for the transaction of business.

Section 5. A majority of the members present shall constitute a quorum of any regular or properly called meeting of the auxiliary.

Article X: Funds

Section 1. All fund-raising activities and subsequent purchases other than regular auxiliary membership dues, shall be subject to the approval of the board of trustees.

Article XI.

Section 1. All documents made, accepted or executed by the auxiliary shall be signed by the president and her representatives.

Section 2. All checks drawn against funds of the auxiliary for routine expenses shall be signed by the treasurer only.

Article XII.

Section 1. The fiscal year of the auxiliary shall commence on the first day of May and shall end on the last day of April.

Article XIII: Parliamentary Authority

Robert's Rules of Order, Revised shall govern the auxiliary.

Article XIV: Amendments

Section 1. These by-laws may be amended by the affirmative vote of two-thirds of the members present, voting at any regular or special meeting of the auxiliary provided the amendment shall have been approved by a majority of the board of directors at a regular meeting of the board, and that notice shall have been sent to the entire membership two weeks prior to the date set for the meeting at which the amendment is to be presented. Such amendment shall become effective on majority vote of the membership at an open meeting.

Home and Hospital Auxiliary
Volunteer's Newsletter

Vol. 1 — No. 1   April

Biggest News of All. An unprecendented first! The public is invited to the institution's first Open House on Sunday, April 26. Hours will be 1:30 PM to 4:00 PM. Volunteers from the auxiliary will be conducting thirty-minute-tours of all facilities: Home, hospital, Forest Park, farm, laundry, etc. Publicity will include guest editorials, press releases, feature stories, and radio programs (on WFAW on April 24 ond 27, 1:30 PM to 2:00 PM). Everyone is encouraged to attend and bring his family and friends. This will be a big project of public information and education. Administrative staff and institution employees, as well as the volunteers, will be working hand and hand in the promotion and production of this event.

o o o o o

Wanted: Members, Members, Members. On March 16 at an open meeting in the chapel, women interested in forming the Jameson County Home and Hospital Auxiliary voted to campaign for memberships. A recommendation of the membership committee was approved, setting $1.00 per day (May through April) as membership dues. It was voted that each person registered as interested in the auxiliary be sent ten registration blanks and be requested to enroll ten more volunteer members. Ten registration blanks are enclosed. **Individuals do not have to volunteer service in order to be a member.** Each pays the $1.00, may participate in in auxiliary meetings, and will receive the newsletter to be kept informed of auxiliary activities and needs.

How to Sign up a Member:

1. One fills out the registration blanks **in duplicate and as completely as possible** gives one copy to the member and retains the duplicate to turn in with the dues.

2. Members who want to work as volunteers on a regularly scheduled basis (once a week, once a month, etc.) mark their preference as to **where** — Home, hospital, or Forest Park. Individuals may sign up for as few or as many hours as they wish.

3. Note preference of any one willing to serve on a committee.

4. One uses the back of the blank to note a particular service or area of interest in which a person is interested or willing to work to use everybody's time and talents **but** use them most effectively. These slips will be the only record of individual preference and interest.

5. New members will be acknowledged and kept informed via our newsletter.

* * * * * *

Next Meeting, Monday, May 18, 1:15 PM at the hospital chapel. New members are urged to attend. Dues and memberships will be turned in. A social get together will follow for a chance to become better acquainted.

* * * * * *

Needed: Officers. Because summer will mean an increase in volunteer activities and because funds are now being received and dispensed, it is urgent that the auxiliary be working within a framework with areas of responsibility and leadership defined. To accomplish this as quickly as possible, it has been recommended that those serving as chairmen of already established committees be elected to serve as a board of directors for one year. This board would then elect its own president, vice president, secretary, and treasurer to serve until next spring. By that time a constitution will be ratified, the needs and services of the group better defined, members will know each other better. This recommendation will be submitted and voted on at the May 18 meeting.

* * * * * *

Committee Chairmen. Members are to encourage others to send ideas and

suggestions to: **Service** — Mrs. ....
.............., Cambridge; **Membership**—Mrs.
........................, Cambridge; **Publicity** —
Mrs. ...., Fort Matkin; **Con-
stitution and By-Laws**—Mrs. ....,
Jameston; **Awards** — **Recognition** — Mrs.
........................, Jamestown; **Entertainment**
— Mrs. ...., Jamestown; and
Finance — Mrs. ...., James-
town; **Temporary Chairman** — Mrs. ....
........................, Fort Matkin.

○ ○ ○ ○ ○ ○

Activity Aide. Are members (or maybe friends) interested or qualified? The
Home is still looking for a full-time activity aide. Her responsibility would be to
work with the county home program consultant and volunteers in scheduling activities and programs for patients in the
Home and Forest Park. Interested appli-
cants should contact Mrs. ....
immediately as the need is urgent. Until
such time as an activity aide is hired,
Mrs. .... will act in this capac-
ity. Suggestions, questions and schedul-
ing volunteer activities in the Home
should be directed to her.

Orientation Sessions. The final session
for Jameson County Home and Forest
Park volunteers is scheduled for April 13,
when work assignments will be made.
Jameson County Hospital volunteers have
had two sessions and will receive on-the-
job orientations this week from Mrs. ....
............................, occupational therapist.
These sessions are designed to acquaint
volunteers with the kind of facilities and
types of people with whom they will be
working. Most comments indicate they
are accomplishing this purpose. The sessions lay a groundwork which makes a
volunteer more effective, and the more
effective she is, the more satisfaction she
gains from the giving of her service. Hats
off to the service committee for getting
our first volunteers off to a well-oriented
start! Everyone "is anxious to get to work."

○ ○ ○ ○ ○ ○

Time Marches on! Summer will soon

be with us and nice weather brings with it thoughts of outdoor activities. The entertainment committee is busy compiling a list of resources (bands, choruses, etc.) which might provide an enjoyable summer program. Who doesn't love an outdoor concert, picnic, ice cream social, or an old fashioned hymn sing? Are there groups or organizations which would sponsor such an activity, send names to Mrs. ...., Entertainment Chairman.

* * * * * *

Orchids. To a group of volunteers headed by Mrs. ...., who provided a glorious afternoon for Forest Park patients! Tea was beautifully served and old fashioned gowns were modeled by the patients themselves. It was indeed hard to tell who enjoyed themselves most, the volunteers who worked, the patients who modeled, or the "guests" who relaxed and enjoyed it all! (See the March 26 **Town and Country Reporter** for pictures.)

To Be Published. A written record of the Jameson County Home and Hospital according to Mrs. ...., has never been compiled. Old records and items of interest are now just scattered in bits and pieces; some are on paper, most are in the minds of elderly board members, trustees, and interested citizens. As a result of current volunteer interest and the pending Open House, a complete history is in the process of being written. Mrs. ...., long-time county home employee and member of the Jamestown Historical Society, is compiling the data. Grandma or Aunt Tillie or Uncle Ned's pertinent remembrances should be shared and sent to Mrs. .... The story is a fascinating one. We've already rediscovered Dr. ...., one of Jefferson county's medical pioneers who, over one hundred years ago, originated legislation for the establishment of our county hospitals based on ideas that are widely held and acclaimed today.

Vol. 1 — No. 2   June

A Home of Our Own The administration has given us two rooms on the second floor of the superintendent's building as a "place to hang our hat." A special committee is now working to make it look and feel like home. The rooms eventually will contain our membership files, records, comfortable chairs, a coffee pot, and a big work table. It will be available for small groups and committee meetings, work sessions, etc. Drop up and see us sometime!

Membership Passes 300 Mark — and is still growing! Enclosed is a membership card which may be carried proudly! Membership is by no means closed. Active members are needed who will give time and service as well as inactive members who will give their $1.00 and will be kept informed via the **Newsletter** published every other month. Dues and the members' names and addresses should be sent to Mrs. ...., Cambridge, Wisconsin.

Charter Officers Elected at May Meeting. Mrs. ...., Fort Matkin, was elected first president of the auxiliary at a meeting in the hospital chapel on May 18. Mrs. ...., Cambridge, is vice president; Mrs. ...., Jamestown, secretary; and Mrs. ...., Cambridge, treasurer. Serving on the board of directors are (superintendent, assistant superintendent, nursing supervisor, OTR in the hospital and activity aide in the Home, and other volunteer committeemen). All will serve an initial one year term.

Get Acquainted Day — July 13. Over fifty new auxiliary members have indicated a desire to become trained volunteers and give service to the Home, hospital, and Forest Park. The original orientation schedule has been revised for a one day super-duper streamlined program which replaces the four sessions held for the first orientation. The day's schedule is as follows:

9:00 AM — 10:00 AM — A special hour session strictly for volunteers, by Dr. ...., Jameson County Home and Hospital consulting psychiatrist. He's terrific—say any of the gals who've heard him! (The auxiliary also invited his regular monthly one and a half hour session with employees.) This will be followed by coffee and a get-acquainted session in the auxiliary rooms.

A noon lunch in the Jameson County Home dining room as guests of the administration.

Tours of the buildings—Home, hospital, and Forest Park. Some of the "experienced" guides from Open House will give a deluxe tour.

Most important: An outline of services, programs, policies, goals and philosophies by the assistant superintendent, Home supervisor, hospital occupational therapist and Forest Park supervisor.

Highlight: Demonstration of "in the ward" and "bedside" games by the activity program consultant, Department of Public Assistance.

These sessions permit one to get acquainted with each other and with people one will be working with. An informed and well oriented volunteer is effective in her work. As a result, she enjoys it more and her enjoyment "rubs off" on the patient. Isn't this really what we're working toward—to have interested, enthused, and as-active-as possible patients?

New Beginnings. We have an impressive list of new projects underway since May:

1. A Bible Study class at Forest Park, enthusiastically received and well attended and scheduled to meet twice a month. (How about leaders for one at the Home and at the hospital?)

2. **A County Home and Forest Park Newsletter** written for and by the residents. Interest and reception has been good with eager contributors; it is expected their numbers will increase.

3. **Chatterbox,** the county hospital newspaper published with a big assist from the patients themselves, typed and mimeographed by volunteers.

4. A leather tooling class in the county home taught by one of our volunteers.

5. First scheduled outdoor band concert and ice cream social to be presented by the Jamestown City Band.

6. A monthly birthday party at the county home and Forest Park. Previously birthday parties were already being held for residents of the county hospital.

Needed: From cellar or attic or "Fibber McGee's closet": looms, sewing machines, records, badminton sets, croquet sets, puzzles, embroidery hoops, needles, crochet hooks, felt and wool scraps, and leather scraps. Such items should be brought to the superintendent's office or one of the officers would pick them up at the volunteer's home.

Orchids and our sincere "thank you" to:

Neil's Print Shop, Fort Matkin, for printing and donating membership cards.

The Bustling Badgers 4-H Club and Jamestown American Legion Auxiliary for the special early June bingo party at the county home. These 4-H'ers are the auxiliary's youngest volunteers and were thoroughly enjoyed by the residents.

Municipal Employees Union 655 for a $50.00 donation.

The Vogue, Geneva's, and Mrs. J. C. .... for beauty shop supplies.

Senior Citizens Club and Episcopal Church for sewing bed pan and pillow covers, bibs, diapers, etc.

VFW Auxiliary for bingo prizes.

Schultz Shoe Factory for leather scraps.

Mrs. .... for sorting and collecting of almost-new used clothing.

The Oakland Ladies' Society for a gift of $10.00 to Forest Park.

St. Paul's Lutheran Church for the use of its mimeograph machine.

·Diamond Oil Company for cones for special summer ice cream treats.

The family of .... for the presentation of a stereo record player for the county home and the administration for a like gift to Forest Park.

The family of Mrs. .... for the presentation of the table lamp for the lobby at Forest Park.

May the number of volunteers already working regularly in the wards rapidly increase!

The Pink and the Blue. Our lovely smocks of pink for the county home and Forest Park, and blue for the county hospitals were purchased and made available by the administration. They were invaluable at Open House for distinguishing our guides. Now they are being recognized by the patients. To the patients the smocks represent "someone who cares," and they've begun to look forward to seeing the volunteers on the wards, in the hallways, and wherever one will be helpful.

Some volunteers have purchased their own smocks—others wishing to purchase their own may do so by contacting Mrs. ...., Jamestown.

Hostess Carts Needed — in the county home and Forest Park. A survey of supervisors shows this to be one of the greatest current needs at the institution. The auxiliary is investigating costs of such carts in anticipation of providing them. This will be a volunteer service bringing items of need and interest to patients in the wards as well as relieving congestion in the superintendent's office.

Almost Ready for Distribution. The first published history of the county home and hospital is at the printers now. Volunteers will be interested in the wealth of factual, interesting and humorous information in the booklet. Mrs. ...., county home employee and former school teacher, did a fine job of research and writing.

Lost and Must Be Found. — Your officers need a contact person in the following communities: Roseville, Ironridge, Morgan's Creek, Lake Louise, Sullivan, and Waterford.

Will anyone interested or who knows of someone who would be interested, please send word to Mrs. ....? Someone is needed to pass information in these communities—and to help make this a true county auxiliary. If one cannot give time as a volunteer worker, perhaps she can help in this project.

Could a Member smile a warm and friendly greeting? Push a wheelchair into the summer sunshine? Take some patients for a drive or shopping? Show family vacation slides sometime? Help with one of the newspapers? Encourage patients to make "scrapbooks" for Central City and Northern Village retarded children? Work with the occupational or physical therapist? Plan an outing to include taking several residents to a community band concert, church social or parade? Conduct a discussion about the good old days or current affairs? Organize a group around a favorite hobby? Interest a 4-H, Homemakers, AAUW, circle, auxiliary, PTA, choir, etc., in presenting a program or touring the institution buildings? Interest a program chairman in a talk about these institutions and the people in them?

If So, We Need You! Contact Mrs. .... or the superintendent's office with suggestions and offers to inform the auxiliary of plans and dates ahead of time.

Attention All Volunteer Workers. Mrs. .... and Mrs. .... met with Mrs. .... at the County Home and Mrs. .... at Forest Park have arrived at the following work schedules for the average week. **(Members sign up to work on the day of her choice.)**

County Home:

Monday: Any craft-work; sewing, bandages, mending.

Tuesday: Shopping for patients; shuffle-board; game day.

Wednesday: **First Wednesday** of month—birthday party for patients, birthdays in the given month.

Second Wednesday of month—bingo games (Prizes are badly needed, as well as help on the second and third Wednesdays.)

Third Wednesday of month—same.

Fourth Wednesday of month—bingo, sponsored by American Legion Auxiliary of Fort Matkin.

Thursday: Card games (prizes neded).

Friday: Help with hair setting; horseshoe games; croquet.

Forest Park:

Monday: Write letters for patients; read to patients.

Tuesday and Wednesday: Take patients for walks; serve pop and popcorn or serve ice cream cones to patients; offer shopping service to patients; take patients for walks or rides.

Thursday and Friday: Help with shampooing and setting hair.

First Friday of every month—help in getting patients to church services and back to their rooms.

Auto rides may be offered to patients at either the Jameson County Home or Forest Park, any of the week.

This schedule was set up to enable a member to decide which day of the week she would like to work, and just where her abilities may be made available.

Suggested prizes needed for bingo are: candy, cigarettes, cigars, small toilet articles (hand lotion, dusting powder, etc.), any stationery, postage stamps; Kleenex; and any small gift items which may be donated.

Auxiliary Meeting. Local papers will give the time and date of the next auxiliary meeting, a meeting held the later part of July; a financial statement will be made at that time.

Thought for the Day. From one point
of view — Governor Dempsey of Connecticut, states: "The world which the young
and the middle aged create for the aged
today is the one in which they themselves
will live tomorrow."

Individual Volunteers

A mature and experienced volunteer may be in charge of small
special-interest groups in the Home, the volunteer selected by
the activity aide as a potential leader adequate to take charge
of a resident group, having proven herself in a probationary period.

On days the occupational therapist in one Home is not on duty,
he leaves for the volunteer, prepared party decoration plans and
patterns with complete directions for her work with residents.
For the individual volunteer who comes Saturdays, the nurse
lists residents who wish to have letters written, manicures, walks
or help in making scrapbooks for children.

Local beauticians donate a day of their time and give women
permanents, set hair and give shampoos. One beautician closes
her shop and brings four other beauticians with her one day a
week. In another Home, a volunteer barber comes weekly to
give haircuts to men.

An auxiliary member regularly escorts interested residents to
a local rural art show of paintings and crafts, exhibits from four
counties. One of the resident-artists, deaf from birth, was especially interested in exhibits having done murals at the school for
the deaf where she once lived.

Those coming into the Home to offer services without "pay"
might be considered to be volunteers; one can say, however, that
the volunteer should never be invited into the Home unless this
service is requested by the administrator or the person in charge;
that the service is needed; and that she is never assigned to work
under an employed person who may resent her or is unfriendly
to her. One has only to put himself in the place of the volunteer
to understand this; ill feeling may result unless circumstances
are exactly right.

Occasionally, a superintendent prefers not having volunteers
in his Home, usually because of some unhappy experience when

the selection of the volunteer was unfortunate or her assignment ill-suited — all as the result of lack of training by the Home. When a request is made for volunteers, someone must be designated by the Home to train and supervise volunteers and to be responsible for their work; volunteers ought not to be asked to register for assignments unless they know who is in charge of the program, since frustration and disappointment will certainly result.

It is not unusual for employees in the Home who have never worked with volunteers to resent the volunteers being given assignments which seem to be "fun" while the employee "slaves" along in humdrum work which appears to be less appealing and is often physically hard.

Prior to requesting volunteers, employees might meet to make up a list of volunteer services which the Home could use as a way for employees to realize their responsibilities in the volunteer program. They consider the reactions of the volunteer working on certain wards with certain illnesses, listing suitable assignments helpful to residents and making preparations along with the activity aide before the volunteer's arrival, considering possible physical risks to her and the resident in the assignment, etc.

The volunteer assignments should always be planned in detail, even before volunteers are recruited; volunteers should be convinced they will be doing something useful — that this activity wouldn't take place unless they were there; that ten residents are now involved in activity whereas the activity aide could only reach four without the volunteers, for instance. Often the activity aide learns a new skill by working with volunteers or assigns them to teach the residents special hobbies or new interests. The volunteers enjoy learning, given an understanding of this service, and enjoy the chance to meet, know and help others, which should be pointed out in recruitment. Again, being useful and needed is important to everyone. One ought to point out, too, that the Home is looking for willing, cheerful, dependable volunteers, nothing more; the Home takes the responsibility of training them and working with them.

But in recruiting volunteers, Homes often discover special talents, useful experience and training in retired people with extra time or den mothers, Sunday School teachers, local artists or musicians. Residents are impressed with volunteers who they know are there because they want to be, are interested in the resident and receive no pay or remuneration.

Volunteers bring a friendliness and devotion often surprising staff and residents. There is no limit to community potentials, potentials which are extending this bridge to the nursing homes from the community.

Volunteers are helping break down the stigmas of old age. Preserving self-respect, sustaining tranquility, and cultivating friendships outside the Home are part of caring for the aged. In recruiting, it ought to be pointed out that one has a great deal to learn from these old people: lessons from their experience and wisdom, stories of historical significance, entertainment in the drama of their lives, patience and courage in facing these last years.

TABLE XII

VOLUNTEER REGISTRATION FORM

.... Home

A. Personal Data

    1. (Mr. Mrs. Miss): ....
                           First Name   Initial   Last Name

    2. Street No. or RFD: ....

       City or Post Office: ....

    3. ....
                     Office Phone   Home Phone

    4. Organizations: ....

    5. Other Special Interests or Training: ....

       ....

       ....

       ....

    6. Car Available: ....

B. Desired Schedule of Services

    1. Contemplated Duration of Your Offer of Volunteer Services:

       1 to 3 mo. .... 3 to 6 mo. .... 6 to 12 mo. .... Indefinitely ....

    2. Time of Day Available:

       Morning .... Afternoon .... Evening .... All Day ....

3. Days of Week Available:
   Sun. .... Mon. .... Tues. .... Wed. .... Thurs. .... Fri. .... Sat. ....

4. Schedule of Visits:
   Weekly .... Monthly .... Twice a Month ....

5. If You Are Available Only at Times Certain Groups or Individuals Are Scheduled, Please Insert the Name of the Group or Individual..................

   ....

C. Areas of Service Based on Interest, Experience or Training (Please Check)

   1. **Recreation:**
      Take Patients for Walks .... Write Letters .... Read .... Visit Wards .... Planning, Directing and Participating in Party Games...........
      Crafts ....
      Can You Play Checkers .... Dominoes .... Pinochle ....
      Rummy .... Cards .... Billiards .... Flinch ....
      Sponsor Parties ....
      Can You: Direct Group Singing .... Kitchen Band .... Play Piano .... Play Other Musical Instrument ....
      Check Hobbies or Interests: Patients' Newspaper ....
      Run a Project .... Nature Study .... Scrapbooks ....
      Others ....
      Active Games: Bowling .... Pool .... Horseshoes ....
      Others ....

   2. **Hobbies**
      Can You Weave .... Sew .... Paint .... Draw .... Clay Model .... Knit .... Crochet .... Woodwork .... Leather Work .... Wood Chip .... Fly Tying .... Rug Weaving ....
      Thread a Loom .... Other Arts or Crafts ....
      ....

   3. **Beauty Parlor**
      Indicate Interest: Give Permanents .... Wash Hair .... Hair Setting .... Manicure ....

   4. **Library**
      Indicate Interest: Reading Aloud .... Library Magazine and Book Cart Service .... Lead Discussion Group .... Library Maintenance ....

   5. **Clerical**
      Indicate Interest: Filing .... Typing .... Mimeographing ....

   6. **Social Service**
      Visit Hospitalized Residents on Regular Basis Who Do Not Have Visitors .... Do You Speak a Foreign Language? .... Which ....

7. **Chaplaincy**

   Indicate Interest: Conduct Bible Reading Classes .... Sing Hymns ....
   Provide Social Atmosphere for Religious Holidays .... Assist Chaplain
   During Services on Wards ....

8. **Miscellaneous**

   Indicate Interest: Receptionist .... Escort Service for Residents ....
   Mending at Home or Church .... Conduct Home Tours .... Furnish
   Transportation for Others .... Furnish Party Treats or Favors ....

List Desired Activity in Order of Preference:

1. ---
2. ---
3. ---
4. ---

Additional Information or Suggestions:

1. ---
2. ---
3. ---
4. ---

State Work or Training which Might Be of Value:

ORIENTATION CLASSES

ORIENTATION FOR VOLUNTEERS ASSIGNED TO WORK WITH INDI-
VIDUAL RESIDENTS. Now that volunteers are recruited and notified
of a date set for the orientation classes, probably held in the
Home, one teaches prospective volunteers their role in the program, describing how the Home operates, how it is financed, its
history, its policies and needs, introducing people responsible for
each area of operation, explaining admissions, and behavior and
attitudes of the residents. The more complete the orientation, the
fewer questions there will be later. Volunteers find that once they
start work, their friends and neighbors will think of them as
authorities regarding the Home, and they should be well informed
to answer the general run of questions the community will ask
about their work.

Orientation includes acquaintance with assignments to be given
volunteers in the Home, as well as some understanding of the
residents and their needs.

The following points may be helpful in volunteer orientation:

1. A resumé of the kinds of illnesses and infirmities of the residents.

2. Preparing the volunteer for the anticipated reaction of the residents.

3. An explanation of the type of activity best suited to various types of infirmities, describing some of the special interests of the residents, specifying the length of activity assignments, and discussion of new activities which may interest volunteers.

4. A tour of the areas in which volunteers will be working — the dining room, recreation room, outdoor areas, and wards.

5. Discussion of any restrictions in working with residents and rules of the Home.

Volunteers ought to have a tour of the Home to find their way around, to learn exactly what is expected of them, what to do in case of emergency, the restrictions, etc. There ought to be an understanding in their orientation, that they are not coming into the Home to be entertained, but that their assignments involve work and often hard work. It is generally discovered that the happiest and most valuable volunteers are those who work the hardest.

Several days of orientation might be given in the Home, or one concentrated day, just as volunteers or the Home prefer. The program which might also serve as a refresher course for experienced volunteers, too, ought to be well planned and start on time, with chairs arranged, coat racks, ashtrays and toilet facilities available, and room temperatures and ventilation properly checked.

A list of questions should be given to each speaker from the Home several days ahead of time, to be answered by him in his talk. This might make speaking easier for him; the length of his talk, perhaps no longer than half an hour, should be designated.

ORIENTATION FOR VOLUNTEERS AS GIVEN BY THE SUPERINTENDENT:

1. The Building.
   a. What is the date of the building and physical changes since that time?
   b. What are some of its interesting features?

    c. How has administrative policy changed during the history of the Home?

2. Personnel.
   a. How are employees hired? How are they scheduled to work?
   b. What are the desired characteristics of the applicants? How are they trained?
   c. What responsibilities do they have in the Home?
   d. What are the duties of the superintendent, matron, charge nurse, attendants, activity aide?
   e. How do they work together? What is meant by OT? PT?

3. Residents.
   a. What are the types of admissions and what is meant by "terminal," "commitments," "ambulatory resident," "senescent patient," "aphasic," "delusional patient"?
   b. What is the approximate number of bed patients, wheelchair patients?
   c. What are some of their infirmities? What is involved in patient bed care? What about surgery services, dental work? What necessary steps are taken when a death occurs?
   d. What are their needs?
   e. What are the nursing standards of the Home? Dietary standards?
   f. What is the mental attitude of the resident entering the Home?
   g. How does the Home attempt to meet his problems?
   h. Are residents free to leave when they like? Who's to prevent their leaving? What are the visiting hours? Regulations for visitors?
   i. What about personal services — haircuts for men, shampoos, manicures for women? Others? How are their shopping needs filled?

4. The Volunteer.
   a. What is the status of the volunteer in the Home?
   b. What help is sought for in the volunteer's services?
   c. What are the obligations and responsibilities of the vol-

unteer taking on her assignment here?

d. What is the responsibility of the Home to the volunteer? What supervision and direction is needed?
e. What is the ideal volunteer like?
f. What are the precautions to be taken in working with the aged and infirm?

ORIENTATION AS GIVEN BY THE NURSE SUPERVISOR:

1. Describe the operation of the nursing service in the Home.
2. Introduce staff or list staff and describe duties.
3. List the illnesses and infirmities of residents: the symptoms, afflictions, treatments, prognoses, dangers involved with disregarding diets, other limitations in their care.
4. How will the nursing service and the volunteers be working together? In what areas will they be restricted? In what ways can the volunteers help? What is the code of ethics in regard to confidences, etc., in the nursing service?

ORIENTATION AS GIVEN BY THE DOCTOR OR MEDICAL DIRECTOR:

1. What are the duties of the medical director?
2. What are the medical standards in the Home?
3. How do these compare with a few years ago, perhaps many years ago?
4. How can friendships help? Visiting? Extra hands and feet? Directly working under certain employees?
5. Discuss any of your personal philosophies in geriatric care, volunteer programs, etc.

ORIENTATION AS GIVEN BY THE SOCIAL WORKER:

1. Job description.
   a. How is one prepared for this work?
   b. What are the social worker's duties?
   c. Why is this necessary to the residents' welfare?
2. What part will social service take in working with volunteers? What supervision and assignments can be expected here?

3. How can volunteers help the social worker?
   a. Exactly how are referrals to be made, for instance?
   b. Examples of situations might be given to illustrate decisions volunteers may have to make in their work.

ORIENTATION AS GIVEN BY THE ACTIVITY AIDE:

1. Description of the activity program.
   a. Why is the program necessary? Describe the values to the residents.
   b. What is the daily, weekly, or monthly schedule?
   c. What attempts are made for reaching each resident through the program?
   What are some of these difficulties, accomplishments?
2. How will volunteers help reach these needs?
   a. How will they be assigned? Will they have preferences?
   b. How many volunteers will be necessary for each assignment?
3. Discussion of the "Do's and Don't's"
   (Typed copies should be distributed and read aloud; sometimes these copies are distributed each time volunteers arrive, are seated, and the list is re-read.)

Volunteers' Rules of Ethics in the Home

1. Leave a resident's room if a doctor comes in to see a resident.
2. Do not enter a room marked "No Visitors."
3. Do not sit on a patient's bed.
4. Consider strictly confidential all information concerning the residents.
5. Report to a registered nurse if any unfamiliar situation arises.
6. Never accept a gift or a treat from a resident.
7. Do not bring treats to residents without approval of the nurse.
8. Do not make suggestions to the residents about certain types of treatment or medication.

9. Do not play favorites. Treat each resident alike.
10. Do not make a promise to a resident that you cannot fulfill.
11. Accept supervision graciously.
12. Do not go on duty with a cold.
13. What you hear should never go out of the building.

SPECIFIC QUALITIES ARE NEEDED IN A VOLUNTEER:

1. Liking for old people.
2. Sympathetic understanding.
3. Sensitivity.
4. Poise.
5. Sincerity.
6. Patience.
7. Cheerfulness.
8. Tact.

To the Volunteer

Volunteer service is a trial experience. After a few hours of service a volunteer who may find herself not adapted to this type of work should not be ashamed or embarrassed to tell the volunteer chairman or activity aide.

There is no distinction between the private paying and welfare patients. Employees do not know who is a welfare resident or who is a private paying resident, and volunteers will not be informed of this confidential information.

Each bed patient has an identification band on his wrist, and the same identification is at the foot of the bed. Additional card information is at the head of the bed, such as special diet, diabetic, forced fluids, to be fed, complete bed rest, etc.

Many patients are senescent who may appear mentally ill, but it must be stressed that senescence and delusions are sometimes infirmities of old age. All the residents are ill physically or they would not be in the Home. The Home is not just a retirement home or room and board home — it is a facility for residents who require medical care or they would not be allowed to enter.

Lastly, a volunteer is not filling the position of salaried

employee; rather she is performing a free, volunteer service as a supplement to the nursing program. The staff is not reduced by the volunteer giving of herself to the residents. Volunteer "pay," so to speak, is in the gratification that she will report to the activity aide in charge.

When coming on duty, one always signs-in at the main office. Each volunteer will be assigned to a specific floor and will report to the activity aide in charge.

RN., Supt.

Do's and Don't's for Volunteers[2]

(Adjustments may be made to the list depending on the Home policies)

Please Remember to:

Be friendly.

Be a good listener.

Obey home rules.

Dress conservatively; use conservative make up; wear conservative jewelry.

Wear low-heeled shoes if possible.

Be prompt in starting the program.

Finish in the allotted time.

Withhold all criticism of the Home.

Act within good taste.

Cooperate with the person in charge of the program.

Refer unusual remarks or behavior to the person in charge of your particular group.

Refer all requests for personal service to the person in charge.

Maintain poise.

Maintain a sense of humor.

Maintain proper attitude toward the aged and infirm.

Use proper speech.

Maintain correct reaction to residents' wants and needs.

Have the ability to control your own emotions.

Act sincerely.

Observe regulations and Home etiquette. Always report to the nurse

Please Avoid:

Appearing to be curious.

Don't discuss patients' illnesses.

Don't handle any medical equipment or personal effects of residents.

Don't give all attention to one or a chosen few.

Don't take anything to residents unless specifically asked to do so by someone in authority at the Home.

Don't sit on patients' beds.

Don't be a sensation-monger.

Don't argue with a resident.

Don't make promises unless they can be kept.

Don't tell an untruth to a resident.

Don't discuss residents or staff on the outside.

Don't make newspaper appeals for recruiting or getting supplies for the Home without permission; such requests and needs must be discussed with the Home and procedures taken for acquisition approved.

Please don't find fault with the physical limitations of working — lack of professional equipment or supplies, card tables instead of wooden craft tables, for instance. The program must constantly ad-on duty before going on the wards. Encourage those residents who do not seem to be actively participating; however, don't be insistent in urging them.

just to cramped areas, just as to other limitations.

Schedules, too, must always adjust to the doctor's, nurses', and residents' schedules, since the care of the resident is of first consideration.

[2] The National Committee for Mental Hygiene: Revised from **Volunteer Participation in Psychiatric Hospital Services.** New York, National Association for Mental Health, 1950, out of print.

IN-SERVICE TRAINING

IN-SERVICE TRAINING WORKING WITH A LARGE GROUP TRAINED FOR INDIVIDUAL AND SPECIAL ASSIGNMENTS. Volunteers are in the Home to be taught; the staff should accept the responsibility of instructing, setting exemplary procedures, pointing out tactfully but firmly, how the activity should be run; behavior or tactics of which the Home disapproves should be corrected immediately, though never in the presence of others. Regulations should be explained again and again, if necessary.

A great deal must be said for the individual volunteer, who can and does give heroically of her time and her love. Red Cross Volunteers often work as individuals having been trained by the activity aide for a probationary length of time under her supervision and direction. As one of the services of the American Red Cross, this agency, upon written inquiry to the local chapter about the needs of the nursing home, will recruit and give some of the orientation required by the Red Cross prior to the volunteers coming to the Home for orientation there.

Individual volunteers are scheduled regularly to work weekly or daily in Homes and hospitals, giving hundreds of hours of work in activity programs, relieving staff who will then have time to develop an expanding recreation program. To express a meaningful life, volunteers encourage residents to do things for the communities, and in nursing homes the volunteers are constantly searching for such projects as will help residents build more useful lives.

A Good Example

In a Home where the activity aide worked with 500 residents in twelve wards, a written request was made of Red

Cross, which recruited and screened seventy-two volunteers to whom they gave a preliminary Red Cross orientation; ten additional hours of orientation were given by the Home. The aide asked for six Red Cross Volunteers to work from 9 AM to 3:30 PM Monday through Thursday. The Red Cross Volunteers came from four nearby cities, a chairman being responsible in each city for having her volunteers working one day a week at the Home.

Six volunteers who reported at 8:45 AM, hung up their wraps, put purses and valuables in a locked room, and were seated while the activity aide read the "Do's and Don't's" aloud, briefing volunteers on anything new at the Home pertinent to their assignments. No other discussion was allowed so there was no wasting of time. The activity aide having worked out schedules with nurses and attendants and having discussed the assignments for the volunteers with the personnel on each ward, would at 9 AM telephone the ward to remind them of the assignment, asking permission to bring the volunteers to the ward.

The activity aide accompanied the group of six Red Cross Volunteers from 9 AM to 3 PM working with them, showing them where to get supplies necessary for the activity, directing them in procedures in coming on the wards; the volunteers learned attitudes and behavior from the activity aide, step by step — how to enter a patient's room, how to deal with his idiosyncrasies and limitations, learning specific interests through which he might best be reached.

The schedule read:

Monday: Volunteers from Lewsville
> 9 AM to 10 AM: Dominoes, checkers, cards, jig saw puzzles, and table games on the ambulatory ward.
> 10 AM to 11 AM: Horseshoes, ring toss, beanbags on men's wheelchair ward.
> 11 AM to 12 AM: Exercises to music, rhythm band with senescent patients in a circle.

Noon
> 1 PM to 2 PM: Visiting, bedside games, and crafts with bed patients.
> 2 PM to 3 PM: Craft shop.
> 3 PM to 3:30 PM: Evaluation of the day, signing up hours served for the day.

Tuesday: Volunteers from New Richland
> 9 AM to 10 AM: Bookcarts on the wards.
> 10 AM to 11 AM: Escorting wheelchairs outside or conducting circle games inside.

11 AM to 12 AM: Visiting and bedside games with bed patients.
Noon
    1 PM to 2 PM: Music Appreciation Class, records, rhythm band.
    2 PM to 3 PM: Craft shop.
    3 PM to 3:30 PM: Evaluation of the day.
  Wednesday: Volunteers from Elmhurst
    9 AM to 10 AM: Discussion class on the wards.
    10 AM to 11 AM: Bowling tournament on the wards.
    11 AM to 12 AM: Assisting people in walking outside.
Noon
    1 PM to 2 PM: Movies.
    2 PM to 3 PM: Craft shop.
    3 PM to 3:30 PM: Evaluation of the day.
  Thursday: Volunteers from Albansville
    9 AM to 10 AM: Wheelchair residents outside.
    10 AM to 11 AM: Table games.
    11 AM to 12 AM: News discussion class.
Noon
    1 PM to 2 PM: Visiting on the wards, guessing contests, drawings.
    2 PM to 3 PM: Craft shop.
    3 PM to 3:30 PM: Evaluation of the day.

What might have seemed an overwhelming job of training seventy-two Red Cross Volunteers then became easy. The activity aide always worked with the volunteers, introduced them to residents and employees on the wards, showed them where games and supplies were kept, helped set up tables and chairs, seated the residents and lead the activity with Red Cross Volunteers and residents. In each instance, she called the ward before starting the activity, and in each instance, stopped briefly to discuss it with the nurse for suggestions or changes for next time. Each time, the activity was terminated ten minutes early to put away chairs and tables, to clean up after crafts or refreshments, with everything in perfect order when the volunteers left the area; volunteers usually shook hands with all residents in farewell.

Before volunteers left, the activity aide discussed any problems or changes which would improve the program, the activity aide always sure they left for home on time, at 3:30 PM, which was the agreement, since volunteers, too, have obligations; usually several volunteers having come in one car would have to leave together.

Red Cross Volunteer chairman in each city in the meantime, continued to send new Red Cross Volunteers, in groups of six each day, for assignments; until finally, after several months all Red Cross Volunteers had reported for assignment in in-service. However, the activity aide continued the same procedure, for months working steadily all day with the six women who came each day, but giving them more responsibility each time, until she was confident things would go along just as well, whether or not she was with them.

Certainly most activity aides have fewer residents to reach, would use fewer volunteers, and work on a much smaller scale, but this type of in-service training has made for a happy, efficient corps of valuable Red Cross Volunteers, giving nearly 600 hours of volunteer work a month. It is possible, of course, for an activity aide not to use any extra time at all in training a few volunteers by having them work along with her for as many times as is necessary for them to learn skills and procedures.

In this instance, the weekly schedule as set up for training was continued, each city group taking the same day, the city Red Cross Volunteer chairman sending the same six women who had worked together and who repeated the same schedule they were originally taught. Finally the six women worked independently, although the activity aide continued always to telephone the ward before the volunteers entered the ward, accompanied them in and got them started, and returned to the ward at the end of the hour to see that they kept their schedule, hadn't forgotten the time, or any details of their leave-taking.

The activity aide was now relieved to branch out into more new recreation ideas, with this multiple assistance going along smoothly. As the year went along and the volunteers gained more and more skill in their original assignment, the activity aide kept two volunteers on the assignment and worked with the four developing another assignment in another ward. Eventually there were three assignments in progress each hour, with two volunteers in charge of each.

Volunteers and staff working together are able to develop programs impossible for the activity aide to do alone. The volunteer can offer her own creativity, new resources, new approaches, and new procedures, with the activity aide's approval. The activity aide is experienced in skills and techniques, but the responsible volunteer can bring fresh ideas that will supplement constructively the aide's work.

Once a new activity is approved by the activity aide, individual volunteers are encouraged not to be afraid of introducing the new idea — perhaps a special interest or hobby of hers which she would like to share with a resident; all is not lost by an attempted activity failing; there is no defeat in having to try again. Often the individual volunteer has the time and patience in urging the resident to do more for himself and more for others, inviting him to the table to watch, urging him to help in distributing the game, bringing up chairs to the tables, working with the visually handicapped or deaf individually and assisting with the party decorations, perhaps.

In the Homes, volunteers are urged to say good morning or to pass the time of day with everyone, whether or not they know the resident, employee, or whomever they meet in the hall.

The volunteer represents the community and the employee or resident, the Home.

A resident says, "Things are a whole lot better since the volunteers are here; we know we aren't forgotten, and things aren't so bad after all."

An employee says, "The volunteers are so helpful — just do anything, so anxious to please; I just couldn't help thinking with volunteers every day, what a wonderful place it is."

VOLUNTEER SUPERVISION

Points in Supervision. Servile tasks shouldn't be meted out to a volunteer, although she should be shown how to put things back in place, sort supplies she is using, all as part of the activity, in working with the employed person responsible; however, she shouldn't be asked to clean out drawers for the staff or sweep floors while the employed person looks on. Common sense tells one that no volunteer is willing to be a lackey for the staff, or should be asked to be.

The activity aide should take the initiative, do the organizing and keep the program within her control always. An activity is never scheduled to satisfy the volunteer's whims; it is the resident's welfare which is considered, working around Home policy and schedules. A volunteer understands and **wants** her assignments geared to the resident's needs, once this is explained to her. Supervision is a continuous thing which establishes self-confidence in a volunteer and utilizes her best capabilities; individual differences should be recognized. The Home must make supervision purposeful in improving job performance, quality and continuity of service. If the activity aide does not keep close contact in supervision, the volunteer eventually gets slack in her work and drops out.

A volunteer isn't recruited to overcome shortages in nursing home staff, but to give a "plus" service, a supplementary contribution. By bringing a volunteer into the Home, the employee is given a chance to give a good impression of it, a chance to show the volunteer the hard-working, able, often dedicated staff she works with and respects.

Volunteers ought to be briefed by the nurse or activity aide on a resident's physical and mental condition, precautions to be taken, simple medication of he is to be gone for some time, and the importance of being near toilets in public excursions or outdoor excursions. Arrangements should be made so that several aides are always in attendance in group affairs.

Residents still feel part of the community if they can attend a local club, school, or church group. A man putting on his best suit, or a woman wearing earrings and perfume, finds life gayer in any age group. Arrangements for church-supper guests sometimes include residents; arrangements for attending the class play given by the local high school are made by the youngsters who escort the oldsters, sitting with them at the performance and giving them a tour of the new school afterwards. A former choir member continues his role by singing in the community church every Sunday, the minister providing the vehicle for his transportation there.

Community groups have reached residents by arranging an exchange of visits with other Homes; the Men's Breakfast Club furnishes transportation, bingo, and the evening meal in an annual outing for the Home, building up a fund during the year for this activity, and meeting with the representative of the local nursing homes to make plans together. A volunteer is appointed responsible for every five residents.

Residents attend an oldtime threshing bee and antique engine show as guests where one of the residents takes pictures of the different types of machines: pump, gas-engine, outside water-cooled tractors, and steamers.

It isn't always possible or necessary to show the volunteer a beautifully equipped Home; but it's important that she see the employees with whom she's assigned doing a good job, whatever the circumstances, and she will be loyal to such a staff.

It is only fair to show a volunteer the "need" and the "know-how," considering her ability and her interest, remembering her time is valuable, too, often necessitating her having to get baby sitters, arranging for transportation, or sacrificing a bridge party, to keep her schedule at the Home.

There ought always to be an optional job offered, so she is never idle, and she ought never to be put in a situation by herself in which she's unfamiliar.

The volunteer should be seen by her supervisor before she leaves the Home to be sure there are no questions, no ill feelings, no misunderstandings; this gives the Home a chance to clear up problems, make explanations, and establish good will.

TEENAGE VOLUNTEERS

TEENAGE VOLUNTEERS, young men and women who have seldom had jobs or been responsible for another person's welfare, find a hospital setting with the aged unfamiliar and need painstaking training and constant supervision. This responsibility must be taken into consideration before they are requested, but many nursing homes have made good use of these extra hands and feet; and their cheerful smiles, enthusiasm, and zip are like a breath of summer. Residents feel flattered that young people like them and that they are willing to take the time from their busy young lives to be with them.

Teenage volunteers are sometimes called Candy Stripers, Pinafores, Peppermint Kids, etc.

Boy Scouts, Girl Scouts, YWCA, Jr. Red Cross, Marias, Mariner Scouts, Boys Brigade, 4H, DeMolay, young people's church

TABLE XIII

RECORDS OF INDIVIDUAL HOURS SERVED

RED CROSS VOLUNTEER SCHEDULE

(Each volunteer has a page in a loose-leaf notebook and she records number of hours served.)

YEAR	1	2	3	4	5	6	7	8	9	10	11	12	13	14	15	16	17	18	19	20	21	22	23	24	25	26	27	28	29	30	31	MONTHLY TOTAL
July																																
Aug.																																
Sept.																																
Oct.																																
Nov.																																
Dec.																																
Jan.																																
Feb.																																
Mar.																																
Apr.																																
May																																
June																																

Year's Total

Name

TABLE XIV

VOLUNTEER HOURS FOR ONE MONTH IN THE COUNTY HOME

Names of individual volunteers under supervision	Apr 1	3	4	5	8	9	10	11	12	15	16	17	18	19	22	23	24	25	26	29	30	Total
Mrs. Henry Larson	7				7					7					7				7			
Mrs. Norman Thomas	3		3				3				3			2						3		
Mr. Ed O'Malley	3			3				2				1			2				2			

groups, and many others, some of whom are given credits for "merit badges," often offer volunteer work and are sometimes more dependable and better organized than scattered groups. Their leader or some dependable adult responsible for them should be contacted in screening them. Sometimes they serve forty-eight hours in a probationary period before being given an arm band, uniform, or badge. A few teenagers assigned to an activity aide may work along with her, learning how to conduct singalongs, games, or outside activities, assisting in craft preparation, delivering supplies to bed patients, escorting wheelchairs outside, manning the record player, etc.

Teenage volunteers are available only during the summer months or weekends and after school during the remaining months of the year, so consideration must first be given their supervision during these times; sometimes the nurse in charge is willing to direct their assignments and be responsible for them after school and weekends when the activity aide is not on duty.

The social worker trained sixty-four teenagers, six of whom reported for work from 9 AM to 3 PM five days a week under her supervision; because of the good training and close direction given them, they became valuable help to the Home all summer.

The social worker said:

My heart sank when they finally reported for work, because I could hear employees along the halls moan when they saw them; they had not been especially useful the year before, running the elevators up and down, laughing loudly; sometimes they couldn't be found at all. There had been too many of them and not enough supervision of jobs to keep them busy. Since this was my first year with them, I was apprehensive.

Employees now are the first to commend them. Teenagers read to residents, wrote letters, served at the reception desk, watered plants and filled water glasses, folded bandages, escorted residents for walks, shopped for them and took them to church, took the bookcart to the wards, worked in the library, brushed and set hair, and gave manicures.

The day before school started they put on a big talent show for the residents, composed songs, and gave skits in costume. They will be brought into the activity program during their Christmas and Easter vacations as a carry-over for next summer's work.

When they left and filled out forms on their assignments, they enthusiastically thanked us for the opportunity of making friends with our residents and being given a chance to help, which was a surprise because we felt entirely indebted to them!

Several of them wrote that they planned to be occupational therapists, beauticians, nurses, or social workers; all of them felt they had benefited by these assignments: "working with people," "learning what sickness meant," "proud of the job we've done." It was a fine experience for all of us, and we're looking forward to another wonderful summer with our teenagers.

Teenage Objectives in Working in Nursing Homes

YWCA: *Pinafores*

Objectives: HOME: To provide some companionship for older people through association with young girls.

YWCA: To provide an opportunity for girls to feel the importance of being needed in the community, and to experience the dignity of service; to understand and appreciate older people; to afford a possibility of future fields of employment.

THE HOME EXPECTS: Compliance with the "Do's and Don't's," the written policies of the Home.

THE YWCA EXPECTS: Orientation and training for girls; progressive areas of service; always under supervision and guidance; candid periodic evaluation with the Y-teen department.

SUGGESTIONS FOR MOTIVATION AND ENCOURAGEMENT: Have consent of parents and willingness on their part for the daughter to give service. Provide some sort of identification, arm band, insignia, smock, etc. Give certificates at conclusion of orientation course, or other recognition for services.

ASSIGNMENTS FOR TEENAGERS: Y-teens will come from the city YWCA to the Home with a service project, on a regular basis. They plan to perform grooming services, bringing their own manicure kits; conducting holiday parties; conducting musical activities working directly with the residents; or in other services to the Home; doing library work; preparing crafts; making posters and bulletin board decorations; and collecting usable items for the Home.

Summer teenagers are assigned mornings in reaching men's groups through games, and giving men manicures. The Home is interested in developing morning activities, a time the assistant superintendent feels residents are more easily reached. Volunteers pass a jar of mints from table to table of residents playing games or working on crafts; a bowl of pansies admired at close range, also makes the rounds enjoyable.

Teenage volunteers show slides in individual rooms, where most of the residents are bed patients or wheelchair patients.

Five large pictures appeared in a local paper showing teenagers reading a Bible passage to a resident, making a tape recording of a blind resident's poetry-reading, playing checkers, posing with residents and their crafts. The newspaper said, "Longfellow Junior High School Junior Red Cross members are no opera stars, but they sing hymns for the elderly at the ————— County Home and Infirmary; they can tell jokes, aid in sewing, push wheelchairs and, in general, make life more interesting for residents there."

A group of three Girl Scouts earned an OTR badge in scouting by making mobiles with residents, working in the Home library, and giving residents rides. A new teenage group has taken over the singing-rhythm band.

Candy Stripers gave a party made possible by the cooperation of the local merchants; the merchant donated candy and pop which the girls sold at a record hop and used the proceeds to finance the party. The girls came early and decorated the living room with a seasonal motif. Three of them, costumed as witches, walked through the halls inviting residents to the party at 6:30 PM, presented a program, and treated their guests to candy from baskets made in their eighth grade school room.

Residents were invited to the local high school for the annual operetta at a special performance given just for them. The auditorium was turned over especially for the occasion, the cast in complete costume, and the band in uniform. This was a great treat for the residents, and for young people, too, who want to know oldsters better. They were given the opportunity to do something for them.

Girl Scout Troop No. 186 named a resident their official grandmother of the troop. A wheelchair resident for several years, her new position was marked by gifts of flowers and plants and "a good supply of her favorite hobby, jigsaw puzzles."

A baseball diamond within a few yards of the Home with a screen for backstop and lights for evening activities is used in a summer schedule of baseball with the city YMCA, a spectator type of activity for residents.

Again, teenagers assigned under the nurses' supervision, come in after school to make down the beds, wash residents' hands and prepare them for meals, fix trays and feed helpless residents, escort them to other areas, supply fresh water glasses, which are changed once a day, wash wheelchairs and medicine glasses, operate the Talking Books record players, and produce a Christmas program.

Girl Scouts come to help make scrapbooks for a local hospital, working in this project with residents who find it a pleasant change from having it done for them. Jr. Red Cross come each Friday afternoon to sew with the Busy Bee Sewing Circle in the infirmary, threading needles, helping in cutting patterns, encouraging, and just visiting.

A county general hospital trained their Jr. Red Cross Volunteers who worked the summer previous as well as each Saturday morning during the school year, in news discussion groups with residents, bowling tournaments, and name-the-tune activities.

A barn at a Farm Home was visited by grade school children, who had never seen farm animals, except on "Captain Kangaroo" or "Carnival" (TV programs), as a way of introducing youngsters to oldsters.

For local Red Cross publicity, the Red Cross Volunteer service was featured in downtown store windows with signs: "Won't You Match Our Dollars with Hours (over 1000) a Year?" Each heart showed weekly hours spent with residents in the county home.

An elaborate and impressive capping service for new Red Cross Volunteers is sometimes held in the Home with residents attending the service, which may include talks by the chaplain, the

TABLE XV

TEENAGER PERMIT CARDS

	CANDY STRIPERS
Name:	
Address:	
Telephone:	
Date of Birth:	

Work days:	Mon.	Wed.	Fri.	Sun.
	Tues.	Thurs.	Sat.	

Number of Hours:

In emergency call:

Date: ....

....

may participate in the Candy Striper Volunteer program at Park
Lawn Home, Green, Wis.

Signature: ....

(parent or guardian)

matron, the Red Cross Field Representative, and the Red Cross Volunteer chairman; there is sometimes special music, lighted candles in a marching procession, and pictures may be taken and a lunch served to volunteers' relatives and friends and the residents in the Home. Especially impressive are the residents filing past, shaking hands with their old friends, the Red Cross Volunteers, smiling, visiting, and congratulating the volunteers.

PARENT'S CONSENT

.... has our permission to work as a volunteer in the .... County Infirmary through the Girl Scout Organization, Riverland Girl Scout Council. It is agreed that the institution will not be liable for any injuries or claims rendered against it for injuries while on duty. It is assumed these will be taken care of by the Girl Scout Riverland Council.

Name ....

Address ....

RECOGNITION OF VOLUNTEERS

RECOGNITION OF VOLUNTEERS. Often, thank you notes to volunteers written by the residents themselves are especially touching in sincerity, extending special sentiment:

Dear .... :

Just two weeks ago tomorrow we had our rug bake-sale. According to Mr. Gowser it was a real success. You helped to make it so by sending out your good coffee cake. This note is to thank you for your help. We would like to have you visit us some day.

Sincerely,

....

Resident's Name
Happy Hours Club

GIFTS FROM THE COMMUNITY

GIFTS FROM THE COMMUNITY. At a Home holiday party, a local
greenhouse sent corsages to women residents attending the formal; formals were donated and men wore white shirts. Birthday
celebrants in another Home receive corsages as gifts from a local
florist each month.

The volunteer coordinator conducted a tour of the buildings
for a group of men from a local church, and shortly thereafter
was notified that this group would raise money to buy a bus for
the institution.

A list posted on the Home bulletin board for volunteers to see,
reads:

> Collect, if you're throwing these things away at home: gift
> ribbon and gift wrapping paper; cloth pieces for stuffed ani-
> mals, quilts, or lap robes; millinery; any items from a sewing
> basket; prizes; cosmetics and manicure supplies: an ironing
> board and irons; greeting cards; square dance dresses; dis-
> carded nylon stockings; rhythm band instruments; writing
> pads and pencils; patterns; neckties. (If they're cleaned and
> pressed they can be used for prizes; if not, they can be cut
> into small squares for a lap robe or pillow.)

Further indication of the interest and love evidenced by the
communities are donations, such as movie screens and community
first-run movies, magazine subscriptions, acceptable clothing;
Christmas gifts or birthday gifts for people otherwise forgotten;
bird feeders or lawn swings; special equipment such as electric
toasters, pool tables or equipment for a carpentry shop.

INSURANCE, LEGAL ASPECTS AND RESPONSIBILITIES

INSURANCE, LEGAL ASPECTS, AND RESPONSIBILITIES. It is important to understand and clearly define nursing home responsibility
for the activity program. It should be clearly understood that the
Home specifies the volunteers' assignments, the duties and time
involved, and the qualifications necessary.

To begin with, it should be determined whether or not the
Home is willing to declare and support measures necessary for
the safety and health of the volunteer. Providing for emergency

first-aid while on duty which is usually given employees, should also be given in orientation class to volunteers. In some Homes, volunteers can transport only residents who have written permits from the nearest of kin, a form filled out and on file in the office; sometimes transportation must be in a Home-owned vehicle with special insurance coverage.

Liability insurance would not be required in states where the Guest Law is in effect: any automobile liability insurance policy covers liability for a "guest," a passenger who is not paying financially for the ride. As long as the driver is not being reimbursed for the trip, her passengers are covered under the automobile insurance policy which the driver carries (see p. 241).

Chapter VIII

ACTIVITIES FOR SENESCENT PATIENTS

We all have a job to help build the ego image. This is very important in the patient motivation. The patient who is dependent, unable to care for himself, eats food that is pureed, drools like an infant and is always dressed in bed clothes, certainly has a crushed self-image. Helping him to be more independent will foster a more wholesome self-image. The self-sufficient individual will be more willing to appear in society and again to be a more normal individual.

EXERCISE CLASS, GOING FOR WALKS OR BEING ESCORTED OUTSIDE IN WHEELCHAIRS.

PRESCRIBED exercises are made by a physical therapist or a doctor since there is danger of a patient overexerting or an injury being inflicted. However, the physical therapist or the doctor often gives the activity aide referrals for games which would be helpful; whether or not the patient should go for a walk or even be taken outside in a wheelchair should be treated in each case on an individual basis and permission be granted by the medical person responsible.

BEACHBALL. Exercise classes are sometimes conducted with an activity aide assisting the physical therapist, or the exercises prescribed by him. Senescent, senile residents or the mentally infirm, seated in a circle, will catch a beachball when bounced to them and begin to laugh, perhaps learning to call another by name as they throw the ball. And whether or not the game is explained to them, they'll catch the ball in a reflex action. If the ball is bounced on the floor instead of thrown directly at them, eye glasses won't be knocked off. Other seated exercises using arms, legs and head motions are given by an activity aide demonstrating in the center of the circle with music; volunteers help the residents, raising their feet or arms as they repeat the motion counting aloud. This type of geriatric patient can be reached sitting in a circle just clapping to music.

SEATED EXERCISES. The following game can be used as a relaxing stunt or as a game of coordination, repeated two or three times, perhaps increasing the speed with each repitition as the resident is able.

Hands on your hips, hands on your knees,
Put them behind you if you please.
Touch your shoulders, touch your nose,
Touch your knees and touch your toes.
Now you raise them up on high,
And let your fingers swiftly fly.
Then hold them out in front of you,
While you clap them one and two.
Your hands upon your head now place,
Then touch your shoulders, next your face.
Raise them high up as before,
While you clap one, two, three, four.

One Home reported the following:

The eleven o'clock senescent group has twenty-two residents who sing as they bounce the beachball or play beanbags, a loudspeaker playing familiar German songs as they sing. The activity aide rings a school bell as the patient makes a target with the beanbag, and for those arms reluctant to rise in throwing, he propels the arms up and down for a few times to start them. One woman able to swing the beanbag back and forth was unable to let go of it, but in two months' time she was able to make a bull's eye; noticeable improvement took place in all the residents — arms and hands were strengthened; there were smiles and laughter. They say, "I wonder what she's going to do now," because there are always some surprises.

Another Home reports, "A doctor who was opening a geriatric unit of 600 beds said, when he saw our wheelchair group of senescents in these circle activities — he could see for the first time that something could be done with these patients."

RHYTHM BAND. Senescent residents tied in wheelchairs to prevent their falling out, often completely disoriented, are difficult

---

' National Recreation and Park Association, 8 West Eighth Street, New York, NY. 10011. **Parties Plus — Stunts and Entertainments.**

to reach; but party paper hats on their heads and a pie tin and wooden spoon in their hands make them feel a lighthearted gaiety that brings smiles. If a record player or a pianist begins some old familiar tune such as a march with a regular beat, heads will nod in time and the wooden spoon and pie tin become rhythm beaters. Triangles or bells, hummers and other conventional rhythm band instruments will add to the tone and may be developed from here.

Discussion. An aide reports on leading a group discussion with senescent patients who seemed lucid about early periods of their lives; discussing some research on the common cold, they remembered treatments for their children's illnesses and could talk about them. Again, they discussed shopping and remembered the marketing of a generation ago. The aide meeting them regularly on the ward starts the discussion by beginning "way back" leading the discussion toward more recent times.

PART II

GAMES AND ACTIVITIES FOR OLDSTERS

Chapter IX

ACTIVITIES FOR BED CARE PATIENTS

*Recognizing accomplishments through physical therapy,
we must say we have only two bed patients, because
everyone is encouraged and urged to get up. They said
when one patient was admitted here, "We've been haul-
ing her stuff around for so long from one hospital and
Home to another, we wonder how long she'll be here";
but we found she needs to have someone to care for. She
needed responsibility and activities where she could take
care of other people, and she's happier here, her family
says, than anywhere she's been.*

REACHING THEM ALL

For craft directions, see "Activities for Residents with Some
Use of Their Hands." For game directions see "Activities for
Wheelchair Residents."

1. Physically Restrained or Disoriented Patients.
   a. Tear rags for rugs.
   b. Fold diapers, napkins, etc.
   c. Knit.
   d. Play with a doll.
   e. Play maracas, tin pans and spoon, triangles.
   f. Color books.

2. Blind Bed Patients.
   a. Make shaggy rugs.
   b. Play coverall.
   c. Sand breadboards.
   d. Refinish or whittle small pieces of wood.
   e. Guess what's in the box, quizzes.
   f. Cut stockings for stuffing animals and dolls.

3. Deaf Bed Patient.
   a. Read.

    b. Sew, crochet, handiwork
    c. Write for the home newspaper or city paper.
    d. Arrange dried flowers.
    e. Do jigsaw puzzles.
    f. Play bedside games.
    g. Paint.
    h. Do quizzes. (deaf patient cited 119 words from the words "Summer Vacation.")
    i. Mend for staff and other patients.
    j. Assemble puppets and other model kits.
    k. Make link belts, leather lacing.

4. Aphasic Patient.
    a. Read or someone read to him (if he can understand).
    b. Do crafts.
    c. Play games.
    d. Have someone give him a manicure, brush his hair; personal grooming.
    e. Study nature.
    f. Watch movies, slides, viewer.

5. Bed Patient with One Hand.
    a. Make pot holders.
    b. Make huck howeling, embroider.
    c. Make link belts.
    d. Make macaroni crafts.
    e. Make gravel mosaics.

Crafts

Salt Clay

Many residents and activity aides have been interested in the crafts of salt clay on exhibit at some of the nursing home workshops — jewelry, decorated place cards, or a piggy bank. Little gifts can be made from salt, water and flour, the "dough" wrapped in tinfoil and kept in a refrigerator for a length of time.

Recipe

1 tablespoon of salt	water
1 cup of flour	a fold of crepe paper, any color

Cut one fold of crepe paper in tiny confetti-like pieces into a large bowl. Add salt and cover with water. Allow crepe paper to soak in water for an hour, or until it is soft. Drain off surplus water, leaving just enough to make the paper moist and pulpy. Remove paper which is for coloring only.

Add enough flour to the colored water to make stiff dough, about like cookie dough. Knead this mixture until is it as pliable and soft as modeling clay. This amount will be enough to cover one small canister, or make any number of smaller items.

Instead of using the crepe paper, vegetable coloring can be used.

Clean and well adapted for bed patient use, this mixture can be worked even with one hand on a newspaper on a bed.

Clay can be colored to match a kitchen and then be used to cover a tin canister in a thin layer, left to harden and dry thoroughly and finally be trimmed with rickrack or gold letters from the dime store; a coat of shellac on the finished product makes it washable.

The clay may be worked with the fingers into petals and flowers and used to decorate a small pin or bobby pin tray; modeled over a small tin foundation, it makes ash trays, which Valspar® varnish will make water- and flame-proof. Modeled over a typewriter ribbon or Scotch® tape box, beads and sequins can be pressed into the clay before it's dry, and when it is dried it can be shellacked.

A can which has a pointed top can be covered with a thin covering of clay after a slit has been cut on one side of the can to make a piggy bank. Decorating it with eyebrows, ears, tail, feet and clay roses makes it amusing.

Copper Foil

Simple 3″ x 4″ copper foil plaques or other items can be purchased for as little as fourteen cents complete and ready to use; a blind person or someone with clumsy hands can make these since it's a matter of rubbing a blunt stick over and over the copper foil on a plastic mold, which improves with rubbing and always turns out well. The necessary rubbing with the blunt stick gives the patient good finger and hand motion. Materials which come with the foil kit include oxidizing, steel wool and lacquer, which a resident may or may not be able to use. The plaque may be framed or can sit on a table or desk as it is.

Pomander Sachet

This is a good craft for a bed patient with the use of his hands. Many patients have made pomander sachets as children to give as gifts: a fresh smelling sachet may be used in a glove or handkerchief box or hung in a closet. It will keep for years. Figure 1.

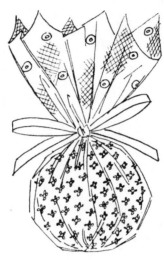

Fig. I

Equipment: An orange or apple; whole cloves; tulle or net 14″ square; sequins; 12″ of ribbon; Elmer's® glue.

Procedure: 1. The cloves are stuck in the orange or apple, close together, until the fruit is completely covered.

2. The orange or apple is placed in the center of the square of tulle and the tulle is gathered together and tied with a bow.

3. Sequins are pasted here and there on the tulle.

Games and Stunts

Icebreakers

When meeting a patient for the first time, it is often easy to start an acquaintance by having something to present in the form of a little game or trick.

1. Ten pennies are lined in a row on a table top. Can the

patient stack them in two's without, in any move, passing over more or less than two cents? Numbering the pennies one to ten, number four goes on one, seven on three, five on nine, two on six and eight on ten.

2. On a sheet of paper, two stars are drawn, one inside the other; the object is to draw a third star inside the two stars (drawing between the two outlines). One must draw it by looking into a mirror set up at the side of the drawing and reflecting the drawing. One may not look directly at the drawing as he makes it.

3. A large letter **F** of heavy paper is cut, as well as its perforated lines, so that it becomes a puzzle, and the resident assembles the **F**. Another letter can just as easily be used, of course. Simple jig saw puzzles can be made by cutting a greeting card, perhaps an appropriate holiday card, into several pieces and the bed patient can then assemble it. Figure 2.

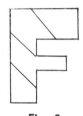

Fig. 2

Rhyme-a-line

The fifth line in these limericks should have as many syllables as the first and should rhyme with the first.

> *All nursing home patients are guys*
> *Who, regardless of shape, sex, or size,*
> *Prefer to eat food*
> *Fried, roasted, or stewed*
> ---.

> *As the barber took up his shears,*
> *He asked, "With or minus, the ears?"*
> *The poor resident sighed,*
> *As he sadly replied,*
> " ---."

In a quiet infirmary ward,
The oldster, to prevent being bored,
Dreamed of beautiful girls,
With lovely blonde curls,

....

Activities for Women

1. RECIPE BOOK: If the resident can cut out recipes from old magazines and paste them in a scrapbook (or on 3″ x 5″ filing cards for a recipe box), she may give recipe books as Christmas gifts.

2. TEA: It's fun watching for the book cart which accompanies the rolling tea wagon, complete with a smiling, dependable volunteer, and talking about the books and drinking the tea she pours.

3. SEWING PROJECTS: There are many jobs for bed patients who will help others: making layettes for needy mothers-to-be; making holiday tray favors, table decorations, cellophane pompons for packages or stitching up mosquito-net Christmas stockings to be filled by a church group or local service club.

It is necessary for the leader to "talk it up," provide the materials and see that the patient's interest continues to make the projects all-absorbing and time-consuming.

Activities for Men

1. SUCTION DARTS: Men with the use of one arm can throw suction darts at the dart board on the wall in front of the bed.

A bull's eye target game is played with a styrofoam ball which a bed patient can throw hitting pointed plastic pins in the bull's eye target which stands in a box at the foot of his bed. A patient with one hand and the use of his arm can manage this and enjoy it.

2. BINGO: A bingo caller in the hallway, a bingo card on a tray in front of each bed patient and a volunteer with each patient to help him cover the numbers as the numbers are called, will bring the bed patient into the game. Numbers will have to be called slowly and repeated.

3. CHECKER TOURNAMENT: An ambulatory resident comes to the bedside to play with the bed patient; the tournament ladder

is posted in each room near the bed where the patient can see the progress of the contest. Residents won't take the responsibility of conducting a tournament themselves, of course; the activity aide or reliable volunter must be there.

For two, three or four players, Egyptian checkers is a combination of checkers and Chinese checkers played on a checkerboard with small colored blocks. The object of the game is to take off one's opponents' blocks and get across to the "pyramid." A score is kept for each block captured and each block which reaches the opposite side. There are advantages in that two, three, or four people can play; the game is easy to learn, and the blocks easy to pick up. The address of the manufacturer is listed.

Concentration Party[2]

1. **Guessing.** The bed patient is asked the following:
   a. Can you guess how many M&M's are in this jar?
   b. Can you guess the number of feet of yarn in this ball?
   c. Can you guess how many pennies can be placed in this medicine glass full of water without making it overflow? The glass, full of water, is placed on the table next to the bed and the patient watches eighteen pennies being dropped into the glass. Many more than one would imagine can be placed in the glass without making it overflow.

2. **Seeing.** A resident is asked to model a new type of wig for the bed patient, the wig consisting of a new mophead with twelve articles tied on it. As the resident turns slowly, all articles are identified by the bed patient. After the wig is put away, the patient tries to name all the articles on the wig: ribbon, can opener, suspenders, scissors, pencil, pack of cigarettes, razor, comb, toothbrush, spool of thread, book of matches and a padlock.

3. **Feeling.** Putting his hand in a ditty bag, the patient feels items he tries to name: pen holder, small bottle, bottle opener, tennis ball, scissors, pack of cigarettes, bag of dried beans, block of wood and a ring.

---

[2] Credited to the American Recreation Society, Inc., **Bulletin.** Ray Butler, Executive Director.

4. **Smelling.** The patient smells the contents of eight small bottles painted or covered with paper to hide the contents; sugar, coffee, tea, pepper, tobacco, candy, soap and face powder, all of which he tries to identify.

Horse Racing Game for Wards

Equipment: 1. One large master track, preferably made from any dark material, the size of the track determined by what would be best adapted to ward participation. A large track covering a pool-table is readily adaptable for recreation hall participation.

2. Small mimeographed tracks, a replica of the master track, for bed patients.

3. Chalk, colored or white, to be used for the master track.

4. Horses; horses from a chess set or bingo numbers can be used.

5. Envelopes containing the number of the horse for each race.

6. Dice, one pair.

Procedure: 1. Each player is given or draws an envelope containing the number of his horse in each race.

2. The game is played with a pair of dice, each dice representing a horse. For example, if one throws a four and a three, horses four and three move one space. If doubles are thrown, then the number of the horse thrown moves two spaces.

3. The tiny squares along the track represent hazards, and a double must be thrown to get over it. For example, should horse number two reach one of these barriers, he may not be moved until two's are thrown. Then he moves into the next space. There are two such hazards on each track.

4. Bed patients follow the movements with colored chalk or colored squares.

The length of time for five races is approximately half an hour.

The reward can be determined by the resources at the command of the leader. As a note of interest, it is found that since participation in the activity may include nearly everyone on the ward, there may be the possibility of a large number of winners in each race; a small prize such as a piece of candy serves very well. As an alternative, prizes could be given on the basis of the total number of races won instead of on an individual basis.

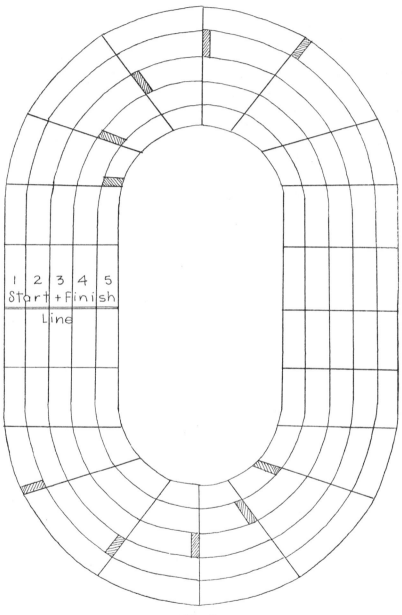

Fig. 3

Hobbies

Birds

Birds offer a variety of activity both inside and outside the Home; very simple or more elaborate bird feeding stations on the window sills or out on the nursing home grounds can be set up for the patient in year round activity. Seeds may be purchased or donated to the Home. Bird books show how to bring birds and how to feed and care for them, as well as including working drawings for making birdhouses, feeding stations, etc. Bird baths will also provide activity, the combination of feeding stations and baths present many opportunities for bird watching for the bed patient. Watching for the first robin in the spring or for each new bird as it makes its appearance can become a game or contest through bulletin board publicity. Roger Tory Peterson's book tells what to look for when identifying birds — What is its size, shape? How does it act? How does it fly? What are its "field marks"? Its voice? Mr. Peterson is the author of **Field Guide to Western Birds** and **Field Guide to Eastern Birds.**

"American Bird Songs," an album of seventy-two bird songs, published by the A. Brand Bird Song Foundation will be helpful in a bird program as a bird call can be identified. There is also an album, **"Voices in the Night,"** by the same company which gives twenty-six frog and toad calls, good activity for the blind in particular. Audubon societies will give information on local bird clubs or list local birds upon request and also serve as a source for volunteer club leaders or speakers.

Gardening

In addition to the usual flower and vegetable gardens, there are also rock gardens, ferneries, herb gardens, wild flower, landscape and decorative gardens and chemical gardens. The local florists or garden clubs will often give seeds in addition to information and advice to the groups. The gardens will provide decorations for the wards and halls as well as for special Home functions. Corsage-making can be added to bed patient activities. Plant pressing may be incorporated into the art and craft program. Since chemical gardening is a relatively new process to most laymen, it might be added that growing plants in water or sand without the use of soil is an interesting venture. Further information can be secured through the Plant Industry Section, University Extension Division, Agricultural Research Administration, U. S. Department of Agriculture, Washington, D.C.

Grass seed will grow sprinkled on a wet cork coaster; lemon, grapefruit, orange pits, radish, pumpkin seeds or beans if soaked in water overnight and planted near the surface of a jar of soil, will begin immediate growth. Carrot or beet tops placed in water with small stones heaped around them make a quick growing garden. A carrot with a well dug in the top filled with water and hung in the window will begin to sprout and become interesting to watch if cared for by a bed or wheelchair patient.

Collections

In old age, people who cannot be interested in starting new collections often revive interest in an old pursuit. Other collectors from the community can do a great deal by visiting with the resident, comparing collections and establishing a friendship through this interest.

Residents leave jars in the lobby for cancelled postage stamps, foreign, centennial, commemorative and different denominations to be sent to a sorting center where they are sold to stamp collectors and the proceeds sent to foreign missions. Many churches will be glad to accept any cancelled stamps of any variety.

SELLING FROM A DISPLAY CASE IN THE ROOM. Greeting cards are sold from an attractive display case in a bed patient's room; in "business" he sells a variety of gifts — silver, ball-point pens, manicure sets, jewelry, aprons, wallets and rain kits. The patient always has visitors; his sales case attracts friends.

Keeping Diaries or Journals; Pen Pals

An eighty-seven-year-old who has kept a journal for forty-eight years, points out a stack of books, two feet high as his journals. Sometimes a person who has shown an inclination in writing can be interested in serving as reporter for the Home newspaper or writing a column for the local newspaper.

Patients like to remember others in birthdays, anniversaries and other holidays; old greeting cards can be cut out with pinking scissors, remounted on typing paper and folded to fit in a new envelope. Many Homes have new greeting cards for residents who want them, the cards often given to them by the local drug store or gift shop as discards following a shop inventory.

Federations of aged people's clubs in foreign lands exchange correspondence with senior citizens groups in this country. Secret pen pals can be found for residents within the Home, and the anonymous correspondents will send greetings. Nonprofit organizations specialize in bringing together adults through correspondence.

WORKING ALONE WITH BED PATIENTS

Activity Aide: I keep several "party boxes" made up with the help of the residents, ready for use with directions for the game, complete with score pads, pencils and prizes. Every time I visit a ward I take a guessing stunt and let the bed patients work on it while I'm doing errands; they look forward to my coming, knowing that I always have something for them.

I've set up a permanent basket with games to be taken to the wards on the spur of the moment from which bed patients can choose; a basket kept replenished — and residents help make these up — with pen and pencil games, quizzes, crossword or nail puzzles.

Craft packets like this could be made with volunteer help, perhaps leaving equipment and instructions on the ward.

Using a magazine picture mounted on cardboard taken to each room weekly, winners guess the identity of the celebrity in the picture, or a song title or a conundrum.

One learns to know the patient by talking to him about anything which might lead to knowing him better and appealing to him. The uniform is a help; they associate the aqua color with activity and when they see me, they begin to ask questions. Sometimes I say, "You'll make me very happy" — the personal appeal, if I'm desperate. Suspense and surprise are good qualities in ward assisting. When they see me come, they say, "What are we going to do today?" because it's never the same thing.

When I was gone for a week, the attendants on the wards

said, "The patients will be so glad to see you — they miss your reading the newspaper to them."

I'm trying to collect stories to send "That's Life" and our local newspaper column "Sam Says," which they read and like. I go on the floors and reach the people who won't or can't come down, and as I read news of their home town I say, "Was she related to the T. L. Smiths? Is that the school across from the creamery? Did your children go to school there? Did you shop in this town? How far is it to Hennepin from there? Is that where the fire was a few years ago? How far was your farm from the church?"

Nurse: Our patients contributed toward cost of the movies and slides from the library — a good way to feel independent and contributing — and we show the movies and slides in rooms; sometimes people feel more appreciative if they have to pay a little for things they enjoy.

We have Talking Book hearing devices, a Sony TV with ear attachment, and our bed patients have earphone plug-ins for use on their beds.

Other residents help aphasic patients in speech therapy as prescribed by the therapist, and some of our bed patients mend hymnals.

Physical therapy is a start in activity; if patients can move around in bed and move their arms and legs, they are more easily motivated, seeing that the activity will help them physically. Patients who couldn't comb their hair or dress get from the chair to the bed and are taught to help themselves. Volunteers can help in the rehabilitative program under direction.

I know their physical strengths and weaknesses well enough to make appropriate suggestions to the volunteers. I stress the positive rather than the negative in everything I say; they keep bringing up the "cloudy day" negatives — I make my visits regularly.

They like visiting with outsiders — children and young people are stimulating, and patients are motivated by simple games, seeing something new, as well as by enjoyment in old familiar things. We ought to talk about new places; these people who have been here a long time don't know what's new. Volunteers should visit regularly.

Chapter X

ACTIVITIES FOR THE VISUALLY HANDICAPPED

Old age is not a defeat; it's a victory.

B<small>LINDNESS</small> need not be totally disabling. Many visually handicapped people, including many who are totally blind, can and do work in the Home preparing vegetables and folding bandages or napkins. Many enjoy recreational activities, the type and extent of their activities, of course, dictated by their interests and their physical capacities. Opportunities for their participation in the Home depends on staff understanding and help.

Blind people may become members of an international club with worldwide memberships, paying annual dues. Hobbyists with tape recorders are listed with their special interests in code, special interests which they may share with a friend in another country; a nonprofit organization, its members exchange tapes they have made.

The following activities are not offered as suitable for all blind or visually handicapped people, but rather they are suggested as types of activities which have proven to be enjoyable and satisfying to some. (The list is not complete in the Appendix, but it is varied and may suggest others.)

Enlarged Print, Talking Books

For those who have limited vision, optical aids are available in many states; by writing the proper agency, Service to the Blind, Department of Public Welfare in one's respective state, help in magnifying devices will be suggested or made available. Division for the Blind, National Library of Congress, Washington, D.C. will give referrals for the nearest state service available.

Current **Reader's Digest, Senior Citizen, Heritage Magazine** and others on tape or records are often available to the aging blind from sources like Aid to the Blind Commission and other state agencies or local libraries. Talking Books are long playing records issued to the Home when the request is made and the name of a blind or near blind person is sent in referral; a representative of a state agency bringing the record player will visit the blind person.

A volunteer can be assigned to play the Talking Books for half an hour to each blind resident, developing discussion following it or organizing a small group of these handicapped people to meet together undisturbed in a quiet room.

People with partial vision, who are unable to read normal size type, may now also enjoy a new special edition of **Reader's Digest** in enlarged type.

Doctors define a "partially-seeing" person as one whose vision cannot be corrected with eyeglasses to better than 20/70 to 20/200 — which means that he cannot see at twenty feet what persons with normal vision can see at seventy to two hundred feet. He cannot easily distinguish the letters comprising normal type. However, copies of magazines are available in giant type, letters two and a half times the size of those in the regular edition (one quarter of an inch high).

The type of reading material should be of lasting interest, non-technical, entertaining, informative and varied in subject matter and very suitable to the aged and infirm. Often, friends and relatives interested in presenting the Home with a gift are looking for something which as many people as possible can enjoy and use indefinitely and would be happy with this suggestion for a gift.

Games

Often blind people who fear failure and lack courage in finding something to do must find programs that minimize aging and blindness. Sometimes physical activity must be restricted, though often residents like to dance, sing, play an instrument, take part in discussions, play cards, enjoy trips and concerts and community affairs, quizzes and other indoor games and contests.

Music often gives blind people a great deal of pleasure.

The blind like team activities with modified rules, bigger balls rolled on the ground instead of batted or thrown, medicine ball or volleyball. One can change the rules of beanbags or ball toss to their use; individual sports like quoits or shuffleboard are easily adapted to each individual. Blind residents play beanbags on the sun-deck, the activity aide directing them to "throw it to me, to the right," or "to the left."

Special cards and games are available from the American Foundation for the Blind, Inc.; all prices include shipping costs; twenty-four cards carry six problems in multiplication and division, a deck of numbered cards in Braille and ink pint; block puzzle, French chess set, plastic checker board, Chinese checkers, cribbage boards, Brailled dominoes, Parcheesi®, bingo, Scrabble®, etc.

In order to teach the blind to use Braille playing cards, the wife of a nursing home manager first learned the necessary Braille herself to make the project possible; she has perforated corners of the playing cards in Braille and then taught those visually handicapped to identify the perforations, a step at a time, first by feeling the position of wooden pegs in similar position on a board. To begin, they started identifying just a few of the cards.

Every day at 11 A.M., five of the blind residents are brought to a quiet recreation area where they sit at a table. They are dealt the face cards and ten of each suit of a deck of Braille playing cards. Residents identify their cards by feeling the Braille and placing the cards on the table as the leader calls them.

"Put out your aces," the leader says. "Now put down the tens; feel across the card from the corner toward the center. Take something else from your hand, and see if you can identify it. No, you're missing a dot."

"That must be a queen," a blind man says.

"Try feeling the other corner, which may not be as worn. Do you have a queen? We're missing one queen. What cards do you have left? That's right! That's a king."

Gradually old familiar games are played, once the cards can be identified. Residents enjoy their achievement, in activity as well as the visits and fun that goes with getting together. Hopefully, other activity will be developed as the group learns these simple skills.

The infirmary has entertained the local White Cane Club, enjoying a weiner roast with them. At meetings conducted by the blind, an interesting flag for the blind was exhibited — the white, satin; the red, velvet; the blue, cotton; the stars, raised embroidery.

Crafts

Basketry may be one of the most satisfactory crafts for the blind, probably the most simple type being the wicker woven into the plywood bottoms which come in kits; one needs a plastic pail to keep the wicker wet, an awl, diagonal cutter, pinchers and the supply of wicker. Baskets can be sold or given as gifts; clumsy fingers find this craft possible since the wicker is large.

The blind particularly like crafts in which they can feel and assemble materials like link belts, mosaics, wood crafts, sculpture and whittling. They enjoy creating pictures by glueing shapes and textures of wood, cloth, wire and plastics on cardboard, constructing cardboard houses or making wood block designs.

Some blind people continue to knit, tat, crochet; others feel useful polishing wood, tearing or snipping old socks for stuffing animals or pillows. Aged people who have been blind since their younger days and have attended schools for the blind often read Braille, weave or continue some mastered skill.

A blind man may turn a handle on a "hobby knit loom" operated by one hand, using broken warp threads to make the ropes which are later sewed into rugs. Hobby knit looms are purcased through craft companies.

After it was said, "You can't get these blind people to do anything," one blind woman made twenty-five disc-dolls and disc-clowns. (Dollie Discs are purchased with directions.) Six blind women sit together every day in the craft room working on these dolls.

A shaggy rug tied on a homemade peach box as a loom was made by a resident who does not see.

Shaggy Rug

This is a good activity for a blind person. Someone makes a simple peach-box loom, prepares the rag strips of material, and sews the rug together for him. This loom makes a usable throw rug or bath mat. (See Figure 4.)

Equipment: Wooden fruit box (peach or apple); two balls of any strong cord; a quantity of washable cloth; five nails and a hammer; scissors; ruler, and heavy button thread and a large needle.

To Make the Loom:

1. One nail is partially driven in the center of the far end of the box.
2. Four nails are driven at the center in the near end of the box, each 2″ apart.

To Prepare the Strips of Rags:

1. Material is cut diagonally and on the bias in strips 5″ wide; these strips are cut crosswise in 1″ strips so that each piece is 1″ x 5″.

Procedure:

1. The resident puts the box on his lap, the bed or table in front of him.
2. He ties the ends of each ball of cord to the far nail securely; he brings cord forward and wraps each around a center nail and to the side nails in a figure eight, to hold the ends securely in place.
3. He places the first piece of cloth over the two cords at the far end, crosses, and brings each end up over a cord and pulls it tight.
4. Each succeeding strip is placed under the two cords, crossed and brought up over each cord. A long strip of shaggy roping will be produced.
5. As the cord is filled with knotted material, it is released from the single nail, extended, and the empty cord is then secured to the nail.
6. When there is sufficient roping, it is coiled, laid flat, the shaggy side out, and the corded side is sewn like a rag rug. It must be sewed flat on a table to keep from buckling.

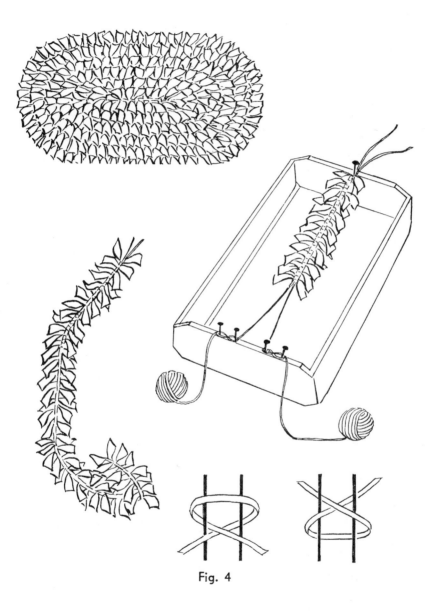

Fig. 4

Chapter XI

ACTIVITIES FOR THE WHEELCHAIR RESIDENTS

We rust out before we wear out sometimes;
I want something to do.
William Koch, Resident

THE GAME and activities included in this chapter are also suitable for ambulatory residents, although they are particularly suited to wheelchair residents. The activities described need not be limited to wheelchairs since, with slight modification, other residents could enjoy them.

ISOMETRIC EXERCISES[1]

Wheelchair bound you say? Can't exercise in a chair?

Residents, whether bed, wheelchair or ambulatory, can increase muscle strength each day. At the beginning or end of an activity, they can do exercises in chairs. Bed patients can do some exercises reclining. These isometrics, pitting of one set of muscles against another, are nine exercises which last six seconds each. By exercising for seventy-two to ninety seconds a day, the muscle strength of most people can be increased from 3 per cent to 5 per cent in a week.

Residents hold their breath while doing the exercise for eight to ten seconds, then relax completely for a few seconds before going on to the next. All nine exercises should be performed every day under direction, doing them carefully, following breathing directions as well as muscle push. In directing isometrics one may find it's better to work individually or with only

---

[1] The Navy: Parade. Parade Publications, Inc., 733 Third Avenue, New York N.Y. Endorsed and approved by Dr. John Allen, MD., Consultant in Medicine, Wisconsin Dept. of Public Welfare.

a few residents at a time. Residents will be able to take the initiative in doing exercises by themselves once they learn them.

A posted sheet on a level where it can be read by resident is a help in following instructions properly:

1. THE HAND PRESS (for arms, chest and shoulders). Sit straight with chest out and arms held across the chest, place one fist inside the other. Press together, using all the strength of the arms and shoulders.

2. THE BACK PULL (for the back). Keep back straight and lean forward until you can grasp your legs or braces of chair. Then pull straight up, using the back muscles.

3. THE NECK PRESS (for the neck). Sitting straight, clasp the hands behind the neck, holding the elbows forward. Pull forward with hands and at the same time press the head backward.

4. TUMMY TIGHTENER (for waist and abdomen). Sitting with legs together straight out, bend forward and grasp the legs just below the knees. Press down with the hands, at the same time press up against the hands with both legs.

5. THE CRISSCROSS (for chest and legs). Placing the feet about four inches apart, bend forward and place hands against inside of opposite knees. Try to press knees together while at same time holding them apart with the hands.

6. THE BODY LIFT (for shoulders, arms and abdomen). Keeping the back straight, lean forward and place the hands, palms down, against the sides of the chair. Hold legs straight out, attempt to raise body about one inch off the chair.

7. THE LEG SQUEEZER. While sitting forward on the edge of a chair, lean back and hold the legs straight out. Hook one foot over the other and hold tightly. Rest feet on floor, keep the legs straight, then try to pull the feet apart.

8. THE ARM CURL (for the upper arms). Sit straight, grasp the underside of a heavy desk or table with palms up, forearms parallel to desk. Push up hard.

9. THE ROPE CLIMB (for arms and shoulders). Clench fists, place the clenched fist of right hand on top of clenched fist of left hand, push up with left hand, down with right. Grasp the

semiclenched fingers of the left hand (palm up) with the semi-clenched fingers of the right hand (palm down) and try to pull apart.

SCHEDULED TABLE GAMES

Since an oldster may not want to play a new game, or is not able to play anything new with complicated rules, sometimes it's best to reach him through playing old familiar games. Volunteers assigned to card tables each having a different game (checkers, cribbage, rummy, canasta, flinch, dominoes, Parcheesi®, euchre and sheepshead) attract the resident to the game of his first choice.

This is an easy way of making friends and may encourage the resident to play later with others once he has found who in the Home plays. Sometimes the staff has found that a quarreling resident is not able to play by himself without a tactful outsider to settle arguments, keep score and keep peace.

Prizes are unnecessary, although one finds that a surprise "drawing," little favors, or a simple refreshment like fruit juice or a drink-mix adds to his pleasure and helps make the activity attractive.

Card-holders often make a card game possible for the resident with only one hand. Three grooves lengthwise in a piece of wood, half an inch thick, about eight inches long and three inches wide, can be used to keep cards upright. A resident can both put the cards in and take them out with one hand as he plays a card game.

Masking tape is used to hold the score sheets or game sheets firmly on the tables; bingo cards with metal windows prevent spilling the markers. Discarded hospital lotion bottles with the tops cut off or paper cups, are used for dice shakers which crippled hands can grasp when a resident can't pick up the dice.

These games can also be played with a bed patient lying flat on his back with a heavy newspaper laid on top of the bed sheet on his stomach, and a shaker and dice in his hand. One must avoid confusing him with rules; the activity aide or volunteer keeps score while the patient shakes the dice until he understands the game.

Once having learned that games can be fun, a few residents

will be ready to participate, and some players will be drawn by curiosity to watch. Most of these games permit the group to expand, and the game is not too badly disrupted if someone leaves. Announcing rules leads to confusion, so rules are given as the game progresses, and the game is started by simply asking the resident to shake the dice.

Because a patient has played a game once or twice does not mean he will remember it a day or a week later, which is one of the reasons a patient is often short with others and an argument can flare up in a moment.

Only after a game has been repeated many times will a player remember the rules completely and so carry a game along once a group is assembled and has started to play. With the leader a part of the group, give- and-take between players is easier; but there will still be many explosive moments.

Good spirits will result as security and success are gained.

A deaf resident need not be excluded from table games; he can play bingo if volunteers will write the number being called in large numbers on a blackboard in front of a table of deaf players.

Coverall is a dice game in which two, three or four people, or a roomful can play; many of these games also can be played at a bedside table with a bed patient.

Coverall

NUMBER OF PLAYERS: Two or more players, preferably not more than four to a table.

EQUIPMENT: Two dice, corn or markers; a card or slip of paper with large numbers from two to eleven.

PROCEDURE: A player shakes the dice and covers the number on his card; he continues as long as he can use the number; when he rolls a number already covered, he passes the dice to the person at his left. The person wins who first covers all numbers in his column.

Letter Bingo

NUMBER OF PLAYERS: Two or more.

EQUIPMENT: Letter dice and long slips of paper on which

is printed a long name, like "Minneapolis," each letter separated by a space. Letter dice can be made of wood, a letter on each side of the dice.

PROCEDURE: As the resident rolls the dice, he puts markers or corn on each letter; he rolls, attempting to cover all the letters in "Minneapolis" before anyone else covers his.

Anyone who can play bingo can play this; what's more, rolling the dice by himself is good hand exercise for the resident.

I Doubt You

NUMBER OF PLAYERS: Two or more; since it is difficult for old people to hold a handful of cards, card holders should be used.

EQUIPMENT: A deck of cards.

PROCEDURE: The complete deck of cards is dealt. The dealer begins by putting face down in a pile in front of him all his aces, saying, "Three aces," perhaps; the player to his left follows by saying, "One one," as he puts down one card, always face down in front of him. The next player in turn puts down two's, announcing as he does so, the number of two's, the next player, three's and so on. Players continue around the table on through jack, queen, king and start over again with aces.

A player may or may not be naming his "lay-downs" truthfully, and he's not required to reveal the cards he's laying down, so they may or may not be what he says they are. If one of the players challenges him by saying, "I doubt you," he must then turn up the card(s) he just played. If the cards are not what he said they were, he must take the challenger's pack of cards and add it to his hand to dispose of. If the cards are what he said they were, he gives his pack to the challenger.

They play until someone gets rid of all his cards and wins.

Help Your Neighbor

NUMBER OF PLAYERS: Preferably three to six players to a table.

EQUIPMENT: Two dice and playing cards.

PROCEDURE: Kings and aces are not used. A deck of playing cards are shuffled and eight cards turned up in front of each player, everyone with the same number, of course.

A player shakes two dice and turns the cards over as he rolls the numbers on the cards; eleven is jack and twelve is queen. The person who shakes a number he can't use, passes the dice to the person at his left, who, if he can use the number, turns the card over and gets the turn; if, however, he hasn't the number or already has turned the card, he passes the dice to his left and so on around the table. The turn goes to whoever can use the number, passing the turn to the left.

If no one can use the number, he continues to shake until he gets what he needs, or until someone at the table can use the turn.

The player who gets all his cards turned face down, wins.

There are many ways of playing, but this is easy and fun for oldsters.

Corks

NUMBER OF PLAYERS: Three to eight.

EQUIPMENT: One cork on a long stout string for each player, a pan top with handle, two dice and twenty-five chips per player.

PROCEDURE: All sit around a table with corks in the center, holding on to the end of the string. The dealer has the pan top and the dice. He has three turns to throw the dice; then the pan top and the dice are passed to player on the left.

The dealer throws the dice; if a seven or eleven turns up, he attempts to put the pan top down on all the corks, while players try to pull their corks away from the center before the pan top descends.

Those whose corks are captured pay the dealer one chip. Those whose corks were not captured are paid one chip by the dealer. A player who jerks his cork out of center on any number other than a seven or eleven owes the dealer two chips. A dealer who claps his pan top down on any number other than a seven or eleven owes two chips to all the players he catches. The game can be played as long as interest continues. The winner is the person having most chips after the original issue is returned.

Card Bingo

NUMBER OF PLAYERS: Any number of players: patients at tables, sitting in ward hallways, or bed patients who can hear from their rooms may play.

EQUIPMENT: Enough decks of cards so that everyone has eight cards.

PROCEDURE: An equal number of cards are turned up at each place, preferably eight. Just as in bingo, the caller has a complete deck of cards, shuffles them and calls them off as he turns them up, "two of spades," "ten of diamonds," "queen of clubs," etc. Players having these cards turn them over; anyone with all his cards turned calls "Bingo." The dealer would do well to arrange the called cards by suits so they can be checked, especially if prizes are to be given.

Bunco

NUMBER OF PLAYERS: One to four people to a table. Opposites are partners.

EQUIPMENT: Bunco is played with three dice.

PROCEDURE: One player at the head of the bunco table rolls one dice; whatever number comes up is trump. The trump number is announced to the other tables, and the play begins. For each trump turned up, one point is counted, except when three trumps turn up at one time when twenty-three points are counted. If three of any other number turn up, five is counted.

Players roll dice until no trump appears; nothing else counts. Head table will call "Bunco" when one set of partners at the table makes twenty-three points. Players at other tables are allowed to make any number of points until bunco is called. High scoring partners are declared winners.

Charge Account

NUMBER OF PLAYERS: Two or more.

EQUIPMENT: Dice with letters, such as can be purchased in "Spell-a-Word" game, or can be made in a carpentry shop. Papers with square marked off four ways are given each player.

PROCEDURE: Dice which represent all the letters in alphabet are rolled and the letters called. Player may write in any letters he wants to use, as they're called. He may not write them in afterward. He is paid $25.00 for every four letter word, $20.00 for every three letter word. Residents will improve after a little encouragement and experience in this game; many of them have seen it played on TV and will pick up the idea easily.

After a designated number of turns, the person with the most money wins.

TABLE XII

$25.00 $25.00

A	C	E	S	— $25.00
	H	A		
	A	C	T	— $20.00
	T	H	E	— $20.00

O Pshaw

NUMBER OF PLAYERS: Three or more, preferably six to eight.

EQUIPMENT: Deck of cards.

PROCEDURE: Cards are dealt until too few remain to make a complete deal. The remaining cards are placed in a pile in the center of the board with the top card turned face up. This card indicates the trump suit.

Beginning with the dealer, each player bids the number of tricks he thinks he can take. A record of each player's bid is kept by the scorekeeper. The dealer leads the suit, and the other players must follow suit, if possible. If unable to follow suit, player may slough a card or play a trump. The player winning the trick leads the next play.

A player can score only his original bid, no more and no less. He scores his bid and ten more. If a player bids zero and takes no tricks, he scores ten; but if a player who has bid zero takes a trick, he scores zero. Failing to make the exact bid, he receives minus one for each trick more or less than he bid.

On the second deal, one card less than the number dealt to each of the players in the first deal is dealt. This procedure is followed until only one card is dealt to each player. Then score is totaled to determine the winner.

Pig

NUMBER OF PLAYERS: Four to twelve.

EQUIPMENT: Deck of cards.

PROCEDURE: The object of the game is to get four of a kind. The dealer deals four cards to each of the players, places the remaining pack face down in front of him, takes the top card from the pack and decides whether he wants to keep the card or pass it on to the player at his left. If he keeps it, he passes one from his hand, calling "Pass." No player must ever have more than four cards in his hand. Each player receives and passes along a card in this manner, all players passing cards at the same time the dealer does.

The dealer continues to take cards from the deck one by one. When the cards again reach the last person, they are piled up beside him, not placed in his hand or used again.

The passing of the cards continues until a player gets four of a kind. He immediately lays his forefinger along the side of his nose, and the players do likewise as soon as they notice him doing this. The last one to perform this feat is penalized by being made one-third of a pig, i.e., being given the letter *P*.

The deal passes to the left for the next hand. Whenever a player is penalized a second time he is given the letter **I**. When he completes the word "pig," he attempts to make other players "pigs" by trying to make them talk to him.

From this point, the game may be played in one of two ways: (a) until all but one player are "pigs," or (b) "hog" or "sow" categories are added and require three penalties each.

Indian

NUMBER OF PLAYERS: Four.

EQUIPMENT: Deck of cards (remove ace, king, seven and two), two dice, prizes.

PROCEDURE: Each person has a complete suit, such as all of the diamonds, etc. All cards are face up in front of the player.

Player shakes dice and turns over corresponding card; if six comes up, he turns over the six of his suit. Jack is eleven, and queen is twelve. He shakes until he shakes a seven, then passes dice. If two one-spot dice are thrown, he turns all cards face up and starts over. If a six is thrown and the six has already been turned, the person to the left gets the turn and may turn his six and so on around. The person to get all nine cards turned down first calls "Indian." When prizes run out, the Indian can choose anyone's prize.

The game is scored by counting five points for each card turned over, plus twenty-five points for "Indian." "Indian" collects all prizes and allows the highest score first choice, second highest to second choice, etc., until prizes are again given out.

PITCHING CONTESTS

Residents are sometimes afraid of feeling ridiculous by engaging in simple contests they think of as childish. The following contests call for little exertion on the part of residents, but skills are required which if done in the spirit of fun, challenge one to make the right response.

Pitching rubber heels at a colorful target, tossing cardboard rings or quoits over a stake or sponges in a wastepaper basket and endless other contests can be adapted for use. Adjusting distances will give the more handicapped a better chance at success; the aide must use individual scores at first with three or four turns to a contest and as they progress, more turns added. The distance may be increased as accuracy develops and the players divided into teams as a last step.

To make an activity more acceptable to residents, one can say, "This is what they do at the church fair concession," and then demonstrate ringing the chair leg with a rope ring, bouncing the ball in the gallon cardboard ice cream container, shooting the bull's eye with a suction dart, throwing the paper plate through the hoop, ringing the neck of the bottle with a ring on a fish pole or dropping the clothespins into the milk bottle.

Or one says, "This is helping your arm, your hand and your shoulder muscles so that you can continue to use them."

Hit Your Home County

EQUIPMENT: A large map of the county or state drawn on butcher's paper and laid on the ground and six rope rings.

PROCEDURE: Contestant has six chances to ring the spot where he was born, for a prize.

There might be larger rings for large counties— smaller ones for those from smaller counties.

Penny Pitch

EQUIPMENT: Card table covered with paper squares, checkers.

PROCEDURE: Contestant is given six chances to toss two checkers completely within squares on card table; cardboard tacked to table edges prevent chips going off.

Sink the Battle Ship

EQUIPMENT: Large tub borrowed from kitchen, pennies and little boats made from paper cups, water and drying cloths.

DECORATIONS: Two stands with signs in shape of life savers: "USS Home" and "Sink the Battleship!" white and blue flags and fringes encompassing the booth; picture of sea in front of the tub; sails on boats painted blue.

PROCEDURE: Contestant attempts to sink the battleship by throwing fifteen pennies in the cup (boat); if he gets five in, he considers boat to be sunk.

Heavier metal discs sink more easily. To make boat sinking more realistic, the contestant must sink the boat before winning the prize, a feat which needs heavier discs than pennies.

Pitching Contests for Holidays

EQUIPMENT: Residents in the craft shop have the teenage volunteers make properties for the pitching contests. (Explanation of the procedure follows "Equipment.")

1. Broom tied to a standard; rope rings.

2. Large skull cut out of white paper glued to heavy cardboard; five pingpong balls.

3. On a white dart-board, a large black owl with white circles around its small black eyes fastened to the board and placed on the floor or leaning against a chair on the floor; five suction darts.

4. A heavy wire circle the size of a basketball goal wrapped with orange paper; five paper plates on which are pasted small bats.

5. A board the size of a card table covered with orange paper and grotesque heads or faces pasted on paper and used as targets; five pennies.

6. A cardboard wheel about twenty inches in diameter painted orange and black, every other number on the wheel with a small witch, bat, owl, cat or pumpkin pasted on it.

7. A five gallon can painted black representing a witch's kettle; six balls of cotton.

8. Two large 3″ wooden dice with black spots large enough to see at a distance; cardboard box.

9. Large orange jack o'lantern posted on a board covered with black paper, large holes cut for eyes and mouth; three beanbags.

PROCEDURE:
1. Ride the Witch's Broomstick — ring the broomstick.
2. Feed the Skull — throw five pingpong balls through open mouth.
3. Hit the Wise Old Owl — throw five darts to hit owl's eyes.
4. Flying Bats — sail five paper plates through a ring.
5. Mask Pitch — throw pennies on paper face.
6. Spider Web — spin the wheel.
7. Stir the Witch's Brew — toss cotton balls in kettle.
8. Lucky Seven — throw dice into box.
9. Pumpkin Throw — toss beanbags through holes.

Once this equipment is acquired, it can be used again and again simply redecorated for other seasons.

Poker Darts

Each card from an old deck of playing card is nailed or thumb-tacked on the wall, wallboard or thick cardboard elevated three feet from the floor or braced on a table. Each contestant is given five rubber suction darts and is told to stand in back of a line a certain distance from the board. The winner is the player whose darts strike those cards making the highest poker hand, five card draw only, of course!

GAMES AND STUNTS

Since games and activities need to be simplified to reach old-sters with handicaps and yet should be acceptable to them as adults, it may help to announce the game or activity with "This is like the TV show." Residents may have seen these shows whose participants they know are "socially accepted, intelligent" adults on TV playing "Password," "To Tell the Truth," "Truth or Consequences," etc. If they still feel that this is an indignity to their adulthood, one ought not to risk the game or stunt, but have another activity ready to try. One must be sure to be laughing with the resident, never allowing anyone to laugh at him.

FILLING CUPS WITH CORNFLAKES. Contestants are shown cups of cornflakes, emptied in a pan. Blindfolded contestants fill the cups with cornflakes from the pan and are told that they must hold the cups over the pan. As soon as the blindfolds are on, however, cups are substituted with the bottom cut out. Pans should be about 8" x 10" to catch the flakes as they fall out of the cups.

FEEDING IN A GROCERY SACK. Large brown grocery sacks with a hole in one side large enough for a mouth are pulled over the heads of two or more men. Blindfolded women are given a banana to peel and feed to the men, who, of course, can't see with the sacks over their heads. The couple who dispose of the banana first, wins the game.

KNOCKING OFF HATS. Spectacles are removed and blindfolds are put on couples who wear paper hats like dunce caps. Blown-up paper bags are tied around the wrists of each person to see who can knock off the other's hat first.

WRAPPING PACKAGES. Shoe boxes are appropriate size items to

wrap; also necessary are wrapping paper cut the right size, and string. Couples compete. Facing one another, two people work together, each using only one hand to wrap and tie the neatest package.

PINNING CLOTHES. Two blindfolded people sit opposite one another, a clothes line stretched between them. Each has twelve clothes pins, and at a signal the contestants pin the clothespins on the line using only one hand. All pins dropped are deducted from those on the line.

TRIMMING HATS. Two contestants with hats, pins, needle and thread and bunches of vegetable or flowers trim the hats in a limited time, then place hats on their heads.

DUCKING CONTEST. Contestants put on a man's derby hat and the leader stretches a piece of string across the room. The idea is to have the contestant try to push his wheelchair under the string without knocking off the hat. He is then blindfolded and the string removed, but he will duck and sway trying to get under the string.

FINDING THE BALL. In a deep box filled with straw or cut-up paper, a small ping pong ball or a very small rubber ball is hidden. A few people, blindfolded, who are given a large pair of gloves to put on, dig into the deep straw for the ball to see who recovers it first.

FETCHING THE FEATHERS. Contestants, who put on gloves which have a little glue on the tips, try to put scattered feathers on the table into two boxes; whoever gets the most feathers in the box wins.

GOSSIPING. One of four residents whispers a bit of gossip to the next who repeats it to the next and so on until the fourth has heard it. He repeats it aloud to see how near he comes to getting it correct or how unlike the original it is.

SHAVING BLINDFOLDED. Ladies lather and shave the men, with safety razor minus blade or a piece of cardboard.

TELLING HOW-TO-DO-IT. A man tells all he knows about baking a cake, and the woman tells about fixing a flat tire.

TRAIN CALLING. Contestants call seven stations in the manner of a train announcer then repeat them with lollipops in their mouths.

BUTTONING THE BUTTON. Two or more persons with a man's shirt and a pair of heavy winter mittens see who can, in the shortest time, button up the shirt while wearing the mittens.

EATING CONTEST. Several couples are blindfolded; at "go" men peel bananas and hand them to the women who eat half while feeding partner other half.

POURING WATER. A cup is placed on the floor; and after each player is given a small pitcher of water, residents pour water into cups. The one who has the most water in his cup has the best nerves.

THREADING THE NEEDLE. Men try to thread a needle in needle threader.

PICKING APPLES. Each contestant picks apples from a basket; the person who holds the most apples in his hands and arms wins.

EATING CUSTARD. Two blindfolded contestants opposite one another, with a dish of custard in front of each, feed each other the custard.

MARSHMALLOW EATING. Blindfolded couples sit facing one another, each feeding the other a marshmallow; first couple fiinishing a certain number wins.

CANE RACE. Canes are set in the ground 8″ or 10″ apart. Each contestant is given four or five wooden embroidery hoops. Taking turns, the contestant pitches the hoop, trying to ring the cane. Prizes may be attached to the bottoms of the canes, or the one hooking the most canes may be declared the winner.

PATCH RACE. After partners are chosen, each women is provided with a piece of brightly colored cloth about 6″ or 8″ square, and a needle and thimble. Each man receives a piece of thread. At the signal, the man threads the needle, and the lady sews the patch on the seat of her partner's trousers. When the patch is securely sewn, they shout to indicate completion.

HIT THE BELL. A bell is suspended in a hoop, and the hoop suspended from a tree or pole. A rubber ball is given the players who take turns tossing the ball, trying to ring the bell in the hoop. One point is scored each time the ball goes through the hoop, and five points if the bell rings.

THREAD THE POPCORN. The object is to see who can string the longest line of popcorn in a given time; each contender is supplied with a darning needle, a supply of popcorn and a yard or so of thread. On the signal, he begins to thread the needles and make popcorn "necklaces." First person finished after three minutes is the winner.

PIPE RACE. Laid out on a table are the bowls and the stems separated from a quantity of corncob pipes, as well as a placement of paper plates with tobacco and a collection of matches. On the "go" signal the contestant picks up a pipe bowl and stem, fits them together, fills the pipe with some tobacco, finds a dry match, and lights the pipe. Whoever sends up the first puff of smoke with a lighted pipe wins.

BEAN ROUTINE. Participant is given a tin cup with a handle, one teaspoon and one cup of uncooked beans; someone holds the mirror high enough so that the player can see himself about 3' or 4' away. Putting the tin cup on his head and looking in the mirror, he dips the contents of the cup in his hand with a spoon and puts it into the cup on his head.

PUTTING ON EARRINGS. Two men are each given a set of earrings, the kind that fasten with a little screw, to see who can fasten a set on the ears of the other first, or maybe it can be his own ears.

"DO THIS, DO THAT." Residents may remember the "Simon says thumbs up" game. Residents imitate the leader in the center of the circle who says, "Simon says thumbs up" and holds up his thumb; but he may try to "catch" them by saying, "Thumbs down" and put his thumbs down without saying, "Simon says thumbs down." Residents who make the mistake of imitating him then are dropped from the game. It's easier to pin a colored tag on people who lose than trying to pull the wheelchair out of the circle to show they're eliminated from the game. The game proceeds with players with no tags.

BUTTON-BUTTON. Playing in a circle with a button on a string long enough to go around the circle, people hold the string in their laps; the button is pushed along surreptitiously by residents with their hands, all of them making hand motions along the string to deceive the leader who tries to guess its location. The person caught with it becomes "it" for the next turn.

HIDING THE THIMBLE. Where could she put it where they

couldn't find it! One of the women hid the thimble three days in her hair, a stunt that makes her a leader in the group. The aide hides the thimble around the room; and even though these people are in wheelchairs, they find it.

IDENTIFYING OBJECTS. "Picnic" involves twelve picnic items each in separate paper bags passed around the circle; residents identify them by putting a hand inside and feeling the fork, rubber weiner, salt, banana, bottle opener, matches, fly swatter, etc.

The game continues with residents writing down three-letter words, taken from the letters in p-i-c-n-i-c. The same idea may be used in "What's in the Christmas stocking?" or anything timely.

TARGET. "Wink the clown" is a game using a picture of a clown with large eyes as a target on the floor into which residents throw poker chips which land on the eye and "close the eye."

TOSSING A HOT POTATO. A player chosen as "it" sits in the center while the others sit in a circle. The players toss a beanbag to one another, making many false moves and gestures. The person tries to touch the bag while it is in the air; and if he does, the last to throw it becomes "it." The passing must not be delayed; the game affords considerable movement.

BALLPITCH. A game is played by residents who throw beachballs in a plastic clothes-basket mounted on rollers adjusted to move in the circle of wheelchairs.

FLAG RACE. Five to ten players are on each team, a large potato for each team is placed on a table on the opposite side of the room, and a tiny American flag is given each player. Players in wheelchairs are pushed up to the table, stick the flag in the potato, and go back to "touch off" the next player.

ITEMS IN CHARADES. Residents may choose important people and describe their names with objects as the following:

> Rockefeller — rock and man;
> Roosevelt — rose pinned on a piece of felt;
> Longfellow — a picture of a tall man;
> Clay — pieces of clay;
> Holmes — pictures of houses;

Shelley — sea shell and E;

Penn — a pen;

Key — a key; and

Bell — a bell.

TEST YOUR SALESMANSHIP. Packages wrapped ahead of time, many of them containing something worthless or comic, are passed one package at a time to music around the circle; when the music stops, the resident with the package moves his chair out and opens the package. When everyone has a package, residents trade packages and give a salesmen's "pitch" for someone benefiting by making the trade. The contents could be a safety pin, a Kleenex tissue, an apple, a bottle top, a plastic strawberry box.

TURTLE RACE. Each resident takes his turn holding the end of a 10' cord strung through a hole in a flat wooden turtle's head. The other end of the cord is attached to a chair leg across the room. Residents compete in urging the turtle to the opposite end of the cord by pulling the cord back and forth. The resident with the best "time" wins the game.

SPELLDOWNS. Since spelldowns seem to put people on the spot when they make mistakes, leaders use mixed letter games with cards on which scrambled words are to be identified and they call it "spelldown."

Other games, such as "go-togethers," mean finishing off what the word on the card suggests: "Meat and ⸺;" "Bread and ⸺;" "Horse and ⸺;" "Coat and ⸺;" "Collar and ⸺," and dozens of others the residents help make up.

"Proverbs" start with giving shortened examples of proverbs: "Lead a horse to water," "Ounce of prevention," etc. Large printed signs give the beginning of the proverb, and whoever can finish the most proverbs wins the most slips. Proverbs on the cards include "A rolling stone ⸺;" "Don't count your chickens ⸺;" "Curiosity ⸺;" "It's an ill wind ⸺."

Games Taken from Radio and Television.

Quizzes done orally are more fun than those that are written.

With "This Is Your Life" each features a brief biography of some club member for the others to guess; residents collect and present this material, the idea taken, of course, from the former TV show.

Games and other TV and radio entertainment are used as ideas for activities which bring residents together daily, sitting in a circle playing the game. As with everything else, the more the participants play, the more skilled they become, and the more they enjoy it. If the game is introduced to them without too many rules, and if the person directing the game thoroughly enjoys it, the patients will enjoy it, too.

"Password" is played with the word "wonderful," for instance, in large letters printed with a marking pen on a large cardboard square and passed around the circle by one of the residents. The panel, or the person guessing, tries giving the synonym as people in the circle, one at a time, give clues — "marvelous," "astonishing," "amazing," "wondrous" until the word is guessed. A group of maximum care patients all in wheelchairs are adept at this game, though they played with difficulty to begin with. They improved by playing it daily and always look forward to the game. There are many other ways of playing — the word may be whispered by someone to each resident, one at a time around the circle, the resident immediately giving a clue to the panel.

"Twenty Questions" is played by dividing one group against another and the leader deciding on some object, a pin someone is wearing, the flag on the flagpole outside, the torch in the hand of the Statue of Liberty; some object they can all locate and are familiar with or can see before them. The leader announces its classification, (1) animal, (2) vegetable or (3) mineral; animal being (1) something alive, vegetable being (2) something growing or that has at one time grown in the ground, and mineral being (3) described as inorganic matter. As questions are asked they are counted, since no more than twenty questions are allowed. The only reply that can be given is "Yes" or "No."

"What's My Line?" has been used by patients guessing former occupations a participant has had; again, if this is played frequently enough, players become skillful and the game goes smoothly.

A nurse says, "Residents play 'I've Got a Secret' and make up a secret. I say to them, 'All of you on pass (a day's vacation) must have done something unusual or interesting.' One of our residents had made a visit to a tree house at her son-in-law's home, a tree house accessible from a second story. Someone else went to a cottage for three or four days where she fried fish, picked mushrooms and cooked outside. This familiar guessing game was fun for everyone and easy for people who watch TV."

TOURNAMENTS

LADDER TOURNAMENTS. The ladder tournament, designed to permit competitive play over a specific time is best suited to Home life of congenial groups, where the players are well known to each other, where facilities are readily available and where there is opportunity for frequent competition. This type of tournament requires a minimum of supervision. It can easily be used for card games, checkers, and croquet tournaments, etc.

TABLE XVIII

Checker Tournament	*Checker Tournament*
1	1 ....
2	2 ....
3	3 ....
4	4 ....
5	5 ....
6	6 ....
7	7 ....
8	8 ....

To facilitate challenges and easy changes of position of players in ladder tournaments, a position board may be constructed in one of two simple methods:

1. Into any 6″ (or larger) board, small nails are driven equal to the number of players. The nails are placed and numbered in order, number 1 at the top. The name of the player can be placed on a small card, circle, or an ordinary price tag. This tag or card may be placed on the nail representing his position in the tournament. Tags can be moved as position of players change thus keeping correct positions of players at all times.

2. If the Home has a bulletin board, a space can be arranged so as to permit numbering in same order as number 1. The names of the players can be put on 1″ x 3″ or 2″ x 6″ pieces of tagboard. Thumbtacks at the ends to hold card in place can be used and the cards moved as the position of players change.

To start a ladder tournament, players or teams can be assigned by lot to a position or placed in the order in which they sign up. The tournament is conducted by a series of challenges. A player may challenge any player above him, not more than five steps up, up to the fifth position of the ladder. Players occupying positions two to five can only challenge and advance one step at a time. All challenges must be accepted and played in order within an agreed time, otherwise the two players exchange positions as though the challenger had won the game. The loser of the challenge must play at least one other game before he may rechallenge the person who moved him out of his position.

The position of each player is constantly posted in order that challenges may be arranged at any time. The final position of each player at the end of the time determines the winner and the position of all other players.

Volunteer men, Red Cross men who have received the same screening, orientation and training as the Red Cross ladies, hold a competitive dart game weekly at a Home, the team from town competing with the team at the Home. Their shouts can be heard coming from the basement to the second and third floors at nine o'clock at night.

Men use a toy pop gun rifle with a cork pellet to hit a pack of cigarettes, a pack of gum, or some other item standing on a shelf at the picnic concession; the gun can't be used for bull's eye practice since the cork flies off a metal target, but it can be used to send a lightweight object off a fence post while the wheelchair residents sit outside, or at the trap shoot meet, winning the object which they hit.

In another Home, women challenge the men to a game of beanbags as a "come-on."

TEAM BOWLING. In the basement of one of the Homes is a regulation scale bowling alley, complete with bowling balls, a pinsetter, scoring table and sheets and chairs for spectators; but in most of the Homes not many residents are strong or active enough to bowl with heavy regulation balls. A game of a portable, light-weight metal rod from which hang five bowling pins, numbered one to five, is easily carried from one ward to another; a team quickly formed comes with bowling sheets, on which the activity aide keeps scores and posts them on the bulletin board. Residents with crutches, canes or in wheelchairs roll a soft rubber ball, half as big as a standard size bowling ball. The fun of competing even though some players are "no good," stimulates cheers and serves as an acceptable "men's activity," familiar yet easy for even the unskilled.

The same type of activity can take place with a bean bag game, the best of which are made in the carpentry shop — a slanting rectangular board braced and set against the wall and four or five medium sized holes with labeled values; rubber horse shoes with suction pegs will hold to any smooth finish floor; rubber darts; shuffleboard (the court is sometimes painted 4' shorter to accommodate this age group); all can be made important and eagerly anticipated if scheduled regularly, rain or shine, developed as a tournament and identified with team members.

This type of activity offers some physical exercise, arm and body movements; but best of all the grins speak eloquently, "It's nice to be up and around."

BUMPER POOL, PIN BALL, TABLE SHUFFLEBOARD, RING-TOSS, BEAN BAGS, DARTS, HORSESHOES AND WHIRLEY BIRD.® Bumper pool, pin ball and table shuffleboard may often be purchased by advertising for second hand machines for sale in bars or recreation halls. People in wheelchairs can and do play.

Rules to ring toss, beanbags, darts, horseshoes, Whirley Bird can be adjusted to rules set by residents and geared to their physical abilities. Ring toss can be made of rope rings and a simple stake made in a stand which will not slide on the floor with suction rubber underneath. Beanbag boards can be made; suction darts should be used in the dart game rather than metal points which are dangerous. Whirley Bird, a game purchased at a hobby shop, has two players each wearing on his wrist like a shield a white disc on which is painted a bull's eye. A player takes turns throwing a suction dart to his opponent's shield, which he catches and scores if the dart touches any of the circles on the shield. This can be played in wheelchairs, since only arm motion is involved.

Playing ball and ring-toss in a tournament encourages activity. A milk bottle on a table of the right height can be ringed as well as the pencil sharpener on the wall or an up-turned chair leg.

Outdoor Games. Badminton has been played in wheelchairs with the net put up between two trees; wielding very lightweight rackets, wheelchair residents intersperse with active teen-agers who play on the team with them.

Jarts, an outdoor game of heavy blunt arrows thrown into a plastic hoop which lies flat on the ground, is easily played even if the weather is windy. This can be purchased at a game or sporting goods store. Tossed like horseshoes, the leaded arrows stand up in the ground landing inside the target ring. The game, the goal of which is the achievement of distance, can be played from a wheelchair. Two or more may play.

An infirmary has a "Wheelchair Croquet Group"; of course, it is necessary to play on cement and to have as many "pushers" as there are players.

HOBBIES

When a leader inspires residents to be interested in hobbies, he ferrets out and brings together a group of people with **special** interests, abilities, backgrounds and limitations.

Everyone is special in nursing homes! The resident is sometimes adversely influenced by his age, sex, ability and interests; that's why one has to be careful to be fair, patient, understand-

Hobbies for Men

Coins
Stamps
Tricks
Puzzles
Model Airplanes
Homemade Games
Knot Tying
Indian Lore and Relics
Cowboy Lore and Brands
Wood Carving
Metal Shop
Wood Shop
Cabinet Making
Woodworking for the Home
  (repairing)
Upholstery
Plastics
Furniture Finishing
Physical Fitness Class (exercise
  games)
Pinochle Club
Checkers
Wheelchair Basketball

Hobbies for Women

Buttons
Dressmaking and Mending
Baking
Knitting and Crocheting
Millinery (remodeling old hats)
Clothing Alterations
Charm Course
Slimastics (exercise games)
Flower Arranging
Slip-covering and Pillow Making
Grandmother's Club

ing, flexible, courteous, good-humored and loving in working with them; nobody must be neglected; nobody should be left out.

One must provide separate activities for special groups, and activities that bring special groups together. They need solo and twosome hobbies, social skills, drama and especially a Home talent project to involve as many residents as possible. They need art in all its various forms. They need someone to play or work with them, accessible areas, relaxed, loving care and teaching of skills.

Hobby Show. A hobby show designed by people sixty years of age or older is given by people who find joy in some hobby, making or collecting something. Golden Agers in the city are invited to display their hobbies with the residents in the Home, and also provide a chance to sell their wares to the public through

Hobbies for Either

Pen Pals
Astronomy and Star Lore
Bowling
Campaign Relics
Chess
Motion Pictures
Adult Recreation (could be any-
    thing new to the resident)
Leathercraft
Golden Age Club
Harmonica Band
Copper Enamel
Pottery (coil or types without
    firing)
Making Tapes of Conversation
Volunteer Leadership Club (resi-
    dents as volunteers)
Nature Hobbies
Piano Requests
World Cultures
Cards
Postcards
Autographs
Paper Maché Figures and Masks

Bird Lore
Felt Craft
Scrapbooks for Jokes, Cats, Dogs,
    Babies and Poems
Hooked Rugs
Wild Flower Scrapbook
Jewelry Making
Painting and Sketching
Ceramics
Creative Writing
Geneology
Fun in Art
Music Appreciation
Choral
Folk Music
Cake Decorating
China Painting
Social Dancing
Sculpturing
Water Color Painting
Little Theatre (reading skits
    together)
Mosaic Tile Work

a selling mart. The show sponsored by the Home is open to the public; there is no entry fee, and anyone over sixty may enter as many items as he likes; every person who enters en exhibit receives a certificate of recognition and a judging committee awards ribbons.

STARTING A SOCIAL CLUB

NAMING THE CLUB. Names for residents' clubs can be determined in a contest run by the residents: The Challenge Club, the Three-Quarters Century Club, the Seniors, Years of Grace, Fascinating World Club, Silver Lining Club, Bright Side Club, The Great Society Club, Blue Jay Club, Live and Learn Club, Thought Starter Club, Opportunity Club, Vagabond Club, Lonely Hearts

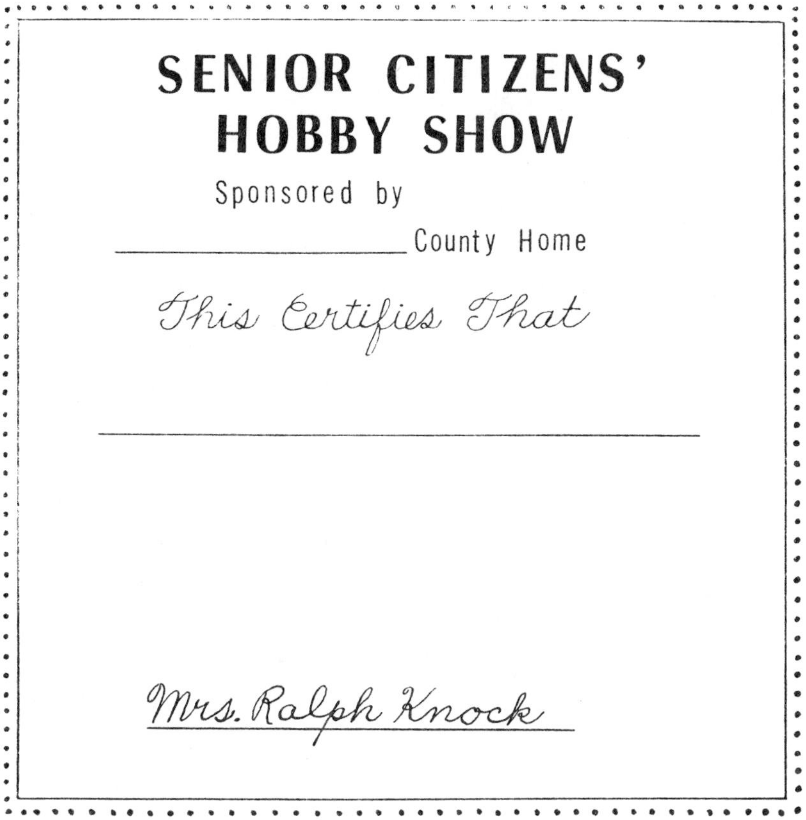

SENIOR CITIZENS' HOBBY SHOW

Sponsored by

_____ County Home

This Certifies That

_____

Mrs. Ralph Knock

Fig. 5

Club, Retirement Club, Strong Shields Club, Comeback Club, Mutual Help Club, Distinguished Citizens Club, Time to Climb Club, Harvest Years and the Plus Seventies. (These are not actual clubs, but only suggestions.)

ATTENDANCE. On a large bulletin board in the recreation room, a resident records attendance; no one wants to see an **X** designating "missing." In other instances a record is kept in the secretary's club record book. Prizes are sometimes given for perfect attendance.

ELECTION CAMPAIGNS. Campaign posters for the election of officers in the club are taped to the walls with enlarged photos of each candidate on the poster. A short catchy phrase should accompany the picture, extolling the virtues of the candidate.

Simple Outline for Conducting a Club Meeting

1. The meeting of the .... Club will please come to order.

2. Will the secretary please read the minutes of the last meeting? You have heard the minutes; are there any corrections? If not, they stand approved as read. (Use gavel.)

3. Is there any old business to come before the club?

4. Is there any new business to come before the club?

5. Will the the treasurer please read his report? Are there any corrections? If not, it is approved as read. (Use gavel.)

6. Will the chairman of the .... Committee
   (name of committee)
   read his report? You have heard the report. Are there any corrections? Any discussions? If not, it stands approved as read. (Use gavel.)

7. The Program Committee will now present the program for this evening. After the program, the meeting is turned back to the president, chairman or leader.

8. A motion for adjournment is now in order. (Use gavel.)

How to Make a Motion

After someone makes a motion, the leader or chairman says, "Will someone please second that motion?" After the motion has been seconded, the leader or president says, "A motion was made by .... and seconded
(name of individual)
by .... that ....
(name)   (subject of motion)
Is there any discussion on the motion? Are you ready for this question? All in favor, please signify by saying 'Aye,' opposed, 'No.' Announce the result. (Use gavel.)

When a member wishes to speak, he should address the chairman as "Mr. Chairman" or the president as "Mr. President." The member must be recognized by the chairman or the president before he may proceed with his remarks.

Ideas for Planning Resident Club Programs (A Home without Volunteers)

A. Call to order.

B. Club song, followed by a "hearty handshake with nearest neighbors."

C. Reports by secretary-treasurer approved.

D. Report of gifts and acknowledgments.

E. Variety of program ideas:

1. Reading of short articles or quotes such as those in digests.

2. Reading of poems, verses from greeting cards or newspaper clippings by residents.

3. Records of favorite music (perhaps keeping time with rhythm band music).

4. Guessing what's in the box, how many beans in the jar.

5. Treats of ice cream sodas or shakes (from the Fun Fund).

6. Music by some local orchestra.

7. Films from the local library.

8. A few dances.

9. Meeting political candidates, since the residents will use absentee ballots for the elections.

10. Residents wearing costumes for special holiday meetings.

11. Children's recitals, dance reviews and school programs given for the residents.

12. Oral quizzes, riddles.

13. Ring toss with scores kept of teams, men against women, one side of the room playing the other, etc.

14. Harmonica, fiddle, or musical saw numbers by resident musicians.

15. Reading Home census of residents a few years back, some still at the Home, of course, and many who have passed on, and impressions of each.

16. Displaying and discussing handiwork in the Home.

17. Introducing new residents.

18. The game of tossing pennies into the muffin pan (around the circle).

19. Songbooks and singing; Mitch Miller record sing-alongs with the sheets of verses.

20. Circulation of special cards or snapshots and greetings to Home residents.

21. Reading excerpts from other county home newspapers.

22. Announcements of new crafts, display of materials; how kits are obtained; costs if any.

23. Dance demonstrations, impersonations, mime, teaching of dance steps.

24. Taking pictures of small groups present.

25. Reading from the Bible.

26. Basketball bounce (into the wastepaper basket).

27. Visits of children just to chat, have a spelldown, recite.

28. Drawing slips and following the directions: "All shake hands and say 'How do you do!' "; sing requested Christmas carols; give a scripture verse; relate memories of other holidays (or seasons); give the names of the books of the Bible starting with each letter in "Near Year" (or the appropriate holiday).

29. Reminiscing (a Christmas forty years ago), reciting a poem the resident knew as a child, vacations: the fourth of July fireworks, the county fair, the baseball lot.

30. Attractively wrapped packages to be passed around and opened when the music stops or used as door prizes.

31. Corsages for the women, boutonnieres for the men.

32. Announcing the arrival of Santa Claus by a fire-truck siren; Santa (or come other surprise guest) distributing sacks of peanuts and candy to the oldsters.

33. "Around the circle" talks from each member who accounts for gifts or mail received, comments on cartoons, radio programs, etc.

34. Stunts (carrying pennies on a ruler, passing pennies around a circle from hand to hand, keeping them moving, feeding one another marshmellows while blindfolded).

35. Playing cards.

36. Reading or telling a favorite joke.
37. A Sunday school class from the community conducting a class at the Home.
38. Contests: blowing the largest bubble with bubble gum; stiff knees, touching hands to the floor.
39. One of the residents giving the history of an approaching holiday.
40. Mixers — drawing duplicate numbers to be matched.
41. Slides or movies taken at the Home.
42. Reading favorite jokes from last Sunday's **Parade.**

F. Announcements.
G. Adjournment.

SOCIALIZING. An activity says:

Start something on a regular basis; begin by singing hymns then socialize. "Why don't we organize a club of rug-makers?" someone says when they receive the first money from making a rug.

I have also been assigned to exercising residents, and this helps getting to know them better, and they know me.

One of our ladies says, "What's today? Monday? Bingo day! I have to put on my brooch and my necklace."

Fannie feels superior to the group because she's a "paying resident" and doesn't come to the meetings; this is what she wants, so we leave her alone.

At our club meeting I suddenly said, "What do you like about the Home? Don't say it unless you mean it!" And the wonderful things each one thought of to say around the circle, were marvelous to hear! We pick up some idea at the meeting, and everyone responds. Some day we may say, "What constructive criticism can you give about the Home?"

We plan on socializing in our club — we sometimes have a meeting with no special activity planned and have some of our best times, everyone just talking together; they love it!

Sometimes I say, "Let's get silly and laugh," and they get a kick out of that — everyone with a different laugh.

I work five days a week, and each day I make contact with each one of our residents. If I'm not here, they wonder why — this is a help in motivation in a club, by getting to know them well through these contacts. I also attend weekly staff meetings with the doctor and nurse; discussing the activity program with them helps because they also work toward motivation.

Types of Social Clubs

The clubs described below are all in existence in various county homes.

THE INVESTMENT CLUB. A county home "Brokers' Office" ventures in "speculation," with the help of a broker-volunteer.

Publicized on the PA system beforehand, the club gives $3000.00 in play money to each resident who cares to participate. All the men and about half the women pick their own companies to invest, and the volunteer helps others. The club shares a brokerage fee and commission like "legit" brokers, and the club brokerage office made $881.00 the first week.

A volunteer purchases a three month subscription to the **Wall Street Journal** to be sent to the Home, and a city brokerage firm sends their tri-weekly newsletter to the Home. The office staff, including the superintendent are stockholders also, often surpassed in success by the resident-stockholders. A graph for each company recording the daily rise or fall of stocks is posted and the club keeps an account book with each member's name, stock-purchased date, number of shares, purchase price, and also a page for the resident's cash accounts.

On alternate weeks each resident is given an additional $1000.00 to invest as he chooses. When he wants to sell, the club purchases the stock at the price that day. One of the residents heard on the radio market report that some company had discovered copper ore on property on which he had stock. The next morning when the **Wall Street Journal** was delivered, he asked the leader to find the name of the company and sold the stock in Ford Motors to be able to buy the copper company stock; but it was a bad move, and he lost in both places.

Each week the leader posts a twenty-four by thirty-six inches chart listing the investors, highest first, to show what each of the "millionaires" is worth. A stock certificate is guarded carefully by residents; dividend checks also designed by residents

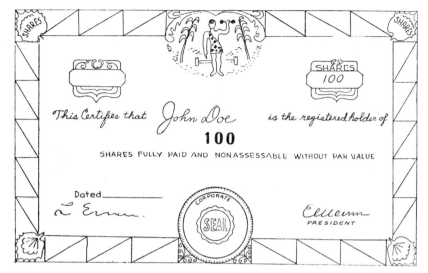

This Certifies that *John Doe* is the registered holder of

100

SHARES FULLY PAID AND NONASSESSABLE WITHOUT PAR VALUE

Dated

PRESIDENT

Fig. 6

pay dividends as the companies do.

One of the residents who had sold his stock when the price had gone up and made $228.00 over and above his fees and commissions asked for his play money which he took to town to show his lawyer. His Greek-English is hard to understand, but he's "wealthy, on top for three weeks running."

The club is well worth the work but wouldn't have been possible without the volunteer, an expert in stocks.

The resident who had earned the most by a certain date was declared winner and taken out to a restaurant for dinner and a night "on the town," the tab being picked up by the Home.

GARDEN CLUB. A local garden club which visits a Home weekly made a fifteen foot oilcloth mural which was hung on a large wall painted with a musical staff, each musical note a picture of birds, insects and flowers. The club conducts discussions with residents identifying each note. The oilcloth simply serves as an attractive way to study nature.

LITERARY CLUB. A volunteer leads residents in a discussion group on familiar, old-fashioned and original poetry, news clippings or verses from greeting cards. This is an important group because it meets regularly.

STORY TELLING HOUR. Held weekly, it involves the activity aide reading an article of suitable length and subject matter from **Reader's Digest** with residents commenting. In another Home the literary discussion is centered around reading aloud from a collection of **Youth's Companion** and other story collections reminiscent of childhood. In each instance the value of the activities lies in the extent in which the residents take part.

A bookmobile which visits nursing homes every three weeks with books gives enjoyment to people perusing the new books. Many Homes have mobile bookcarts on the wards and new magazine racks complete with plastic covers protecting new magazines.

SPORTSMEN'S CLUB. Men residents listen to games and reports over the radio, learn names of players, keep records of scores of baseball, football and bowling games which they watch on TV, making scrapbooks of players. Is there a nearby college which will be willing to plan a bi-weekly game night or a tumbling exhibition? Officers and committees in the club can be formed, and swapping yarns is a favorite pastime of "old cronies." Opportunities for fishermen to talk to fishermen and hunter to hunter rekindle old interests. Baseball prediction contests are a natural consequence during the baseball season; preparing a list of answers from the Sunday paper and correcting the sheet takes very little time; still it's fun.

LEAGUE OF WOMEN VOTERS. An interesting project resulting from a book review by the city League of Women Voters has developed into a league unit of twenty resident-affiliates in the Home. Men and women residents may join the league as active members taking on full responsibilities in dues, leading in discussing and electing officers with full league privileges; subjects introduced by the club have been water conservation, foreign policies, health, Latin America and Cuba.

A unit of twenty members of the League of Women's Voters was set up in another Home. Residents followed the discussion and study plan which they conducted with help from community league members assisting with study materials.

MONTHLY SUPPER CLUB. This project was developed by twenty-four residents attending the craft area classes who voted on having a supper prepared by themselves for a few guests; residents voted on the date and on a menu with many things from which to choose. A resident committee made the cheese sandwiches which were then dipped in egg batter and fried by the president (sitting in his wheelchair and wearing his beret) for the forty residents and guests at a supper club meeting.

The residents invited the guests, made the place cards from old greeting cards and put up the forty foot banquet table outside the craft area; two men in wheelchairs who set the table served as an entertainment committee. Committees in table decorating designed a large cardboard lion and eight cardboard lambs set in stands and placed as intervals down the length of the table and arranged a spring bouquet for a centerpiece.

Especially noteworthy in this distinguished group of eighty-year-olds was their industriousness and sense of responsibility, their adequacy in introducing guests and visiting together, one of them saying the blessing, another the benediction at the end of the meal. (A hard working cleanup committee member said confidentially, back of hand, "They couldn't get along without me.") Guests included the superintendent, some of the attendants and other employees and other residents in the Home, the minister and his wife and the county home program consultant.

Getting dressed up, bathed and shaved was all part of the day's excitement and drew the suspense of the month's planning to final achievement and a pleasant satisfaction in their weariness. These are people with handicaps in wheelchairs, without good muscular control, with paralysis and crippling; some of them are deaf or unable to speak — but they show their colors and they are a credit to their Home. Best of all, they help publicize the activity program, making it attractive to other stay-at-homes on the wards.

The Monthly Supper Club business meeting includes having the minutes read and new minutes recorded.

"I don't want to be on the committee — I like no one and no one likes me," one of the men had said at a first meeting; but it's interesting that, put to a vote, only two residents agreed to "let him off the hook."

THE MERRYMAKERS. At a residents' club in a Home with

seventy-five residents, fifteen of the thirty-five residents attend club meetings in wheelchairs.

The first gathering of residents was in the living room with the attendant who had been assigned an eight hour afternoon shift as activity aide to "tackle" a huge pile of hospital gowns and residents' clothing to be mended. Every Thursday afternoon or evening all through the summer, get-togethers were growing more popular, and song fests, games, a talent show and a rummage sale of good-as-new used clothing, accessories, jewelry and cosmetics donated by friends entertained them.

At a meeting in September the possibility of organizing a club was discussed. A key resident was named president, who suggested the name "The Merrymakers of Happy Acres" for the club, and composed words for the theme song to the tune, "The More We Get Together." Another key member entrusted with funds from the rummage sale was appointed secretary-treasurer, and the activity aide was elected vice president with thirty members enrolled and no dues charged.

The aims of the club were to get acquainted, form a closer relationship among the residents, promote good fellowship, have fun and relaxation, and perhaps discover some latent talent. It has done all this and more, like one large family developing a spirit of cooperation, friendliness and responsibility for the well-being and happiness of others.

Each meeting is brought to order at the rap of the president's gavel and opened with the club song accompanied by hand clapping. The minutes and financial report are read by the secretary-treasurer, and seconded for approval; announcements are made, followed by the program. Everyone is encouraged to take part around the circle; members, in turn, contribute a reading, tell a story, joke, riddle, recitation, song or some interesting event in their lives, giving residents confidence and experience in self-expression.

Games have not only provided fun and exercise but also have developed alertness and muscular coordination. A popular feature is guessing what's in the mystery box, which contains something edible which is also the prize. The "Fun Fund" supported by rummage sales and voluntary contributions from residents and friends outside the Home furnishes treats or a lunch often partially prepared and served by residents. The rhythm band, suggested by a member who was a former music teacher, has developed, each resident having kitchen "instrument" to play a rhythmic beat to the accompaniment of either of the two pianists in the group.

GOLDEN AGE CLUB. Membership in a local Golden Age Club which meets in the Home has advantages to the residents in meeting here rather than in town; often residents are overly tired after a trip into town and three or four hours in a crowded room. Also, many more residents can enter into the club activities if it's held in the Home, going back to their rooms as they become tired. Other clubs such as the local pinochle group, checker club or any card club meeting at the Home can easily encourage residents in a game; a volunteer sitting at a table is always a special attraction with an invitation for them to sit down and play. Some Homes encourage local talent; play groups give dress rehearsals in the Home or provide a practice room for the local barbershoppers.

SPECIAL INTERESTS

Discussion

Procedure in Remotivation

In the May, 1962 **Reader's Digest,** leaders of a specific technique, remotivation, tell of the therapy developed by a volunteer in hospitals in which conversation, sometimes just a word or two, may eventually reach a withdrawn patient, stimulate him and bring him back to reality. This technique is a therapeutic treatment medically prescribed; but everyone enjoys it whether leading a "normal" life in a busy, productive world or living in a nursing home, where this type of "cure" is not a goal but a pleasant stimulating pastime.

In many nursing homes, activity aides or the social workers in the Home, in one instance two Red Cross Volunteers, have had a thirty hour training in which they work with patients and gather material on twelve topics of interest to the aged and infirm. Once this material has been compiled — pictures, poetry and items to model, pass around or display — the activity is set up, and the aide is ready at the drop of a hat to reach for the folder and take charge of a session.

REMOTIVATION SESSIONS IN NURSING HOME PROGRAMS.[1] Remotivation is a technique for use by a trained aide. A part of good nursing care, the technique is supervised by professional nurses. The aim of the program to "remotivate" patients to take renewed interest in their surroundings is by focusing their attention on the simple objective features of everyday life. At the same time, remotivation encourages the attendant to take a more personal interest in his patients.

Today there are over 11,000 nurses and aides and at least 90,000 patients participating in remotivation programs in hospitals and nursing homes.

The program is sponsored by the American Psychiatric Association and is administered and financially supported by Smith, Kline and French Laboratories. An APA Advisory Committee supervises the program and continually reviews established policies.

The technique of remotivation consists of a series of patient meetings held once or twice a week under the leadership of an attendant or a trained volunteer. Usually the series consists of twelve sessions, with each meeting lasting from thirty minutes to an hour. In each group there are from ten to fifteen patients who are encouraged, but not required to attend.

The attendant initiates a discussion, purely objective in nature, by using as conversational material such things as current events, history, natural history, geography, national holidays, etc. The sessions give even the most regressed patient an opportunity to enjoy something with other people even if his pleasure is limited to the sounds and rhythms of poetry, a friendly smile and a pleasant voice speaking to him. The hope is that this technique will remotivate the patient — get him moving again — in the right

---

[1] Further details about The Remotivation Technique are available through
　　　　APA/ Smith, Kline and French Laboratories,
　　　　Remotivation Project, Box 7927,
　　　　Philadelphia, Pennsylvania, 19101

direction. Remotivation is a structured program which permits the attendant to plan his material based on five specific steps. The steps involve "Creating a Climate of Acceptance" for the patient, "Building a Bridge to Reality," "Sharing the World We Live in," "Developing an Appreciation of the Work of the World" closing with "A Climate of Appreciation."

CHIT AND CHAT. Over forty-five residents have signed up for nothing so technical sounding as a weekly Remotivation Class, but a "Chit and Chat." Classes meet weekly to discuss "sports" in which they show a surprising amount of interest and information in university rulings, scores and scope of events; at a following class about "The Old-fashioned Kitchen," they discussed the pump that had to be primed, the bucket that went down in the well to keep things cool, the old coffee grinder and the wood stove.

The activity aide, in passing around pictures of old-fashioned ice boxes asks, "How did you get the ice? Where did the door open? How are new refrigerators different? Are there some advantages? Is refrigeration really important? Do you remember the names of some of the old ice boxes? The new refrigerators?"

With the resident reminded of a joke or a recently forgotten experience he wants to tell, reminiscing and carried away, he is also learning and sharing. The leader makes a point of accepting whatever comment the resident wants to make; no criticism is ever given of an answer or a right to answer it. The resident is accepted for what he is and made to know he is loved. He may digress, disagree, prove unpopular, biased or libelous, but he is always accepted by the discussion leader.

In one discussion class with "Fashions" for the subject, the residents were surprised and excited by witnessing the array of old-fashioned ladies' clothes complete with underwear, which a staff member modeled. In another class an item like a sea shell — "Where did it come from? What do you really hear now? How is it formed? Ever been to the beach? Tell us about it. What is a chambered nautilus? Can you tell about some other forms of sea life?" — can lead to forty-five minutes of comment. The leader goes from one person to another in a circle, bending close so he can hear, and asks the questions, to the right and left and back to keep them contributing, interested and taking part.

One sees in this class people who are actually waking up; one sees new animation, questioning, assertions of self respect, a reincarniation of independence and renewed dignity leaving the class still chatting and interested in being included in the next meeting. This is a good carryover activity developing growth, charting incentives in listening and contributing and "belonging to the group."

In one of the nursing homes, the four trained activity aides who conduct residents' classes, train ward attendants in the Home in a week-long course in understanding the program showing how they, too, can continue these discussions informally with residents on the wards and in their rooms as they work. Nurses find activities of this sort invaluable in giving residents a new lease on life since the residents do less quarreling among themselves, actually complain of fewer aches and pains, are less dissatisfied and lonely, make new friends and find new interests and learn to socialize and express themselves, being proud of taking part.

It is easy to start with a small class, maybe six accessible residents; hearing seems to be the only prerequisite in joining a discussion; one reads an article on a subject in which residents would be interested and collects some pictures which might be helpful to pass around the circle. Sessions should never be longer than forty-five minutes and perhaps this first one should be even shorter. The class should suggest the subject for next week, at the same place, same time; they're off to a lot of fun with a most valuable activity!

Below are some suggested subjects for "Chit and Chat":

"Scares I've Had"
"My Most Unforgetable Character"
"Things I'd Like to See Again"
"Places I'd Like to See Again"
"If I Were to Write a Book, I'd Tell . . ."
"My Favorite Picnic"
"My Favorite Carnival"
"The Worst Winter I Ever Remember, the Hottest Summer"
"The Person to Whom I Owe the Most"
"The Best Neighbor I Ever Had"

ArOUSING CONVERSATION. The activity aide rouses conversation with the simple query, "What would you do if you were in the park and someone fainted?" They say, "I'd set him up." "I'd put water on his head." "I'd lay him flat on his back." "I'd telephone for someone."

"Who would you call? Where would you find a telephone?" These questions can lead to other areas of discussion.

Sometimes the activity aide reads something from "In Uniform" in the **Reader's Digest** and before finishing reading the anecdote asks, "What would you have done?" to encourage comment. Another reads a "Dear Ann Landers" or "Dear Abby" letter without reading the answer and asks each resident in the circle how he would answer it.

If residents can wear clothes that are respectable, they will have more respect for themselves and others; if they feel they don't look well, they won't want to be seen and they won't want to be heard. They want to know that someone is interested in them, so one gets them to speak. Old friends may mean a great deal to old people with something to talk about so they will keep in touch.

QUESTIONS FOR THE DISCUSSION. A discussion group, perhaps sitting outside in a circle, one afternoon a week, talks about the "Old-fashioned School" as the activity aide asks questions around the circle:

> What was the first school you remember? Anyone remember a sod building, adobe or log? What color was it? What was the floor like? The heating? Who kept the fire going? How far did you have to walk? Were you ever given a ride? What do you remember about your first day of school? Your lunches? What were the games you played at recess? How many children in your school? Do you remember anything unusual about families attending? How many months a year was school held? Do you remember the school picnic? What did you have to eat? What was the entertainment? What about Christmas at school? What training did your teacher have? How was she hired? Have any of you taught country school? How old were some of your youngest teachers? Was arithemtic taught differently from now? Spelling? Reading? Do you remember the names of some of your readers? Do

you feel schools lacked a great deal in those days? What benefits would a child of today have in school? What's happened to the one-room schools? Why, do you suppose? Do you remember any tragedy happening at your school? Anything especially funny? What were some of the contributions of the old-fashioned school? Was more, or less, emphasis put on ethics in those days? Religion? How have modern science and modern gadgets changed the needs in the old curriculum? Do you remember some great teachers in your youth? How did they influence you? What are some things you're glad you don't have to live over, in the old-fashioned school? What were some of the hard things in life then?

The subject for next week should be determined; residents will certainly have suggestions so the subject can be announced for the following week.

"Work I Did as a Young Person" might be used asking each question again and again around the circle:

What were some unusual jobs you've had? Perhaps the women will remember unusual jobs in housework if not in a profession, or unusual jobs their husbands had. How did you get your training for these jobs? Have some of you learned your jobs in another country? How would that job compare with this same work today? Is there a living to be made in your job today? What was your first pay? What were living expenses like, compared with the job? What was rent? Taxes? Clothing expenses? Cost of food? Did you have any vacations from your job in those days? Would you choose the same job again? What did you enjoy about it? What was unpleasant or hard? If you were choosing a job today, what would you like doing? What would you find tedious? What would you especially appreciate in keeping house today? Are any of your grandchildren, nieces, or nephews following your footsteps?

"Strangers Who Used to Come to the Back Door." What experiences have you had with gypsies telling your fortune? Selling things? What do you remember about their dress? How did they live? How did they travel? How did your people feel about them? What do you remember about tramps? Do you remember any scares in your community as a youngster? What was the life of a tramp like? Do you have any Indian stories? Experiences as children? What were these people like? Do you know any Indian lore, traditions, superstitions? What prejudices did your family have about these people? Do you think their precautions were well-founded? What were peddlers selling at the back door in those days? What companies did they represent? As a child, how did you feel about strangers? How did the peddlers travel? What were distances like in those days? How did news travel then? Do you remember instances when news traveled slowly? Did your family ever give people at the back door, work? Have you ever been lost, or for some other reason, gone as a stranger to someone's back door?

"What Travel Used to Be Like." Did you ever have a runaway with a horse? Have you heard of such accidents? What used to frighten a horse? Horse thieves are sometimes compared with automobile thieves today; how were horse thieves apprehended? How were they punished? What were trains like in those days? How old were you before you ever left the boundaries of your county? What was the longest trip you've ever taken by horse? By train? Do you remember your first ride in a car? What kind was it? What made travel in a car less attractive than it is today? How much walking have you done in your day? What do you think about the 50 mile hikes? Did some of your ancestors travel in covered wagons? Have any of you flown in a plane? What are your impressions of that kind of travel?

"The Old Circuses." Do you remember your first circus? Have you seen a circus unload? What can you tell us about it in detail? The kitchen, the dining areas, the dressing rooms, the care of the animals in traveling? What were some of the funniest clowns you've seen? Have you seen disasters from storms during a performance? Accidents? Have you known people who traveled with circuses? What were the old-fashioned circus parades like? Have any of you visited a Circus Museum? What animal acts did you especially like? Were there animals you disliked or feared? What sensational side shows do you remember? Concessions? Games of chance?

Talking Book Discussion. Talking Books from Aid to the Blind are really records which may be used to develop discussion; in one Home, eight visually handicapped people sit together with a volunteer each Monday morning and listen to the record which they use as a basis for discussion.

In another Home, residents meet daily in the lounge, one of them in charge of the record player in a "Chapter a Day" group.

News Discussion. Some Homes subscribe to the grade school senior **Weekly Reader** or other grade school newspapers to which a local school subscribes; a copy comes Mondays, little sheets in large print of current national news, which is read aloud by the group of residents around the table. Questions following the articles are discussed together. For five dollars, twenty residents are supplied with an activity for five months.

Wheelchair Square Dancing

Wheelchair patients who were once old-time square dance fiddlers, callers or dancers may especially enjoy being pushed to a square dance call.

1. The Home ought first to purchase a record player and records. The records should be music without the square dance calls, but to which square dance calls could be given. The records with calls are too fast.

2. Arrange for a room large enough for eight wheelchairs moving about in square dance formation.

3. Schedule a time and arrange for eight volunteer square dancers or employees in the Home who know square dance calls and one of them who can "call" the formations.

4. Place two wheelchairs to the north side of the room, two to the south, two to the east and two to the west, all facing the center and assign a pusher (a volunteer square dancer) at the back of each chair. As the record plays, the caller calls the formations; each pusher follows the directions by pushing his wheelchair through the dance.

Residents whether participating in wheelchairs or as spectators love to shout out and keep time clapping, swinging and swaying.

Virginia Reel[1]

This is done to the music of the Virginia Reel.

---

[1] Don Brick, Recreation Agent, Walworth County, Elkhorn, Wisconsin.

Formation: Double line of chairs facing each other. Three or four pairs to a set.

Allow enough room between chairs so that "dancers" can pass each other easily.

Allow enough room in aisle between partners for reel.

Action: All chairs forward and bow (back to place).

Forward and right wheel round (place right wheels side by side and pivot around and then back to place).

Forward and left wheel round (same as above with right wheels).

Forward and dos-a-dos (partners pass each other on right and go around each other back to back).

Head couple forward and turn one and a half times round (place chairs with right wheels side by side and pivot one and a half times).

Head couple "wheel" (reel) (partners split and go to first chair on opposite side and pivot left wheels).

Back to center and pivot right wheels with partner (continue pattern until partners reach end of line — then partners again pivot one and a half times and move side by side back to original position).

Lead them around (head couple turns to outside and wheelchairs up to opposite end of the line — other chairs follow, pass through the former head couple and re-form lines with new head couple).

Repeat until all couples have served as head couple.

Take a Little Peek

Music: "Irish Washerwoman" or other square dance record without call.

Formation: Square in couples (lady always to the right).

Action: Designates couples 1, 2, 3 and 4 in counterclockwise manner.

First couple out to couple on the right. (First couple wheels out in front of second couple.)

Round that couple and take a little peek. (First couple splits and goes and peeks behind second couple.)

Back to center and swing your sweet. (First couple comes back to center and pivots with right wheels together.)

Go around that couple and peek once more (same as before).

Back to center circle four. (All four chairs circle in clockwise direction until couple two is in center, then couple one passes between couple two and on to couple three.)

Repeat above action with couple three and then couple four.

This entire process is repeated with all four couples.

Holding an Auction or a Rummage Sale

Nursing homes which have been given donated clothing and other useful articles might, during a recreational period, use these items for a rummage sale. It is a treat, indeed, for shut-ins to go on a shopping spree and be able to handle and select from this used but good-as-new merchandise, many "bargains grabbed up for a dime."

In raising money, residents like the idea of having a Chinese auction, bidding a penny up to the highest bidder; in a "silent auction" a resident writes his name and the amount he would bid on a slip of paper which he places under each item, the item going to the highest bidder.

One of the residents, a former auctioneer, prints and posts bills, giving time, terms and a list of items for the sale. He also serves as a good auctioneer.

A Home wrote a nationally known celebrity (TV or movie star) for some cast-offs, perhaps clothing, which could be auctioned off as a way of raising money for an activity fund.

In a basement storage room, under the supervision of two women in the main office, the Home sold women's articles on one side, men's articles on the other. On one side were dresses hanging on a long pole, a box containing other pieces of clothing; on a table were handbags, jewelry, thread, handkerchiefs and shoes. On the men's side were hats, suits, jackets, ties, sweaters and pipes. Residents were allowed to try on the clothes before buying them.

Music

Community Sings on the Wards

Almost everyone of every age likes music, whether it's keeping in time with noise makers, listening to live music or recordings, or actually singing. Volunteers sometimes have conducted church choirs or children's singing groups and find directing community sings easy in the wards; occasionally an inexperienced person with a strong singing voice directs a group and if no accompaniment is available, a leader with a strong voice may be successful alone.

Old people lack singing volume; but they are proud of being in a Home chorus, whether it's formally scheduled and developed in part-singing or just a cozy, congenial group around the piano warbling hymns and old songs at their request.

It would seem that the old-fashioned singing films, with the bouncing dot touching each word as it's sung would be useful if the films could be rented. Lantern slides flashed on the screen are effective too.

One of the best songbooks found was purposely printed for aged singing groups in nursing homes, the print half an inch high.

MUSIC APPRECIATION CLASSES. In some Homes, music appreciation classes are developed with the attendance recorded. "We use volunteers to 'man' the phonograph reading aloud and discussing the description on the back of the record album. Good albums, we find, are old familiar ones such as **"Sing Along with Mitch"** and we ask, 'Do you remember what was going on when this was popular?' and we reminisce similar to the former 'That Wonderful Year' TV feature. We play 'Baby Face' and then ask, 'Anyone remember someone who had a baby face?' ' "Now is the Hour" — when was that popular?' We take residents up in their wheelchairs, and the men are 'hosting' the women; next week the women 'host' the men, standing at the door to welcome them. Sometimes we discuss the composers of Strauss waltzes and semi-classics. 'Carousel' and 'Oklahoma' are popular music with this group. Volunteers have donated all the records we use. We have typed the words to songs so that we can play the record and sing it using these typed sheets."

Sometimes residents have sketched or doodled as they listened. Another music appreciation class has just meant playing "oldies" on a record player in the hall for bed patients who could sing along or make requests from their rooms. Sing-alongs have become popular with TV shows and are more easily conducted now that residents have seen them. There are a number of song games such as "give the next line," "identify the tune," or "make up stories using the names of songs." Usually the most popular music are waltzes or old-fashioned songs easily identified. A former music teacher can add a great deal to the group; and again, a group that meets regularly becomes an important group.

INDIVIDUAL MUSICIANS. Former organists, music teachers and professional musicians are residents in almost every Home, along with amateurs who enjoy playing an instrument. A weekly Home talent show is presented with residents who give readings, sing, tell jokes, even do sleight of hand tricks. Little skits and jokes of the old vaudeville type are presented with the resident dressed in a donated costume reading the lines in front of the mike.

MUSIC FROM THE COMMUNITY. Residents in one Home enjoy the visits of seven county Golden Age groups who come in on a regular basis with song fests, plays, accordian music, an octet, the Sweet Adelines and the Barbershoppers with community sings, etc. A Home plans folk dances every two weeks with residents taking part.

The concert given by the Baraboo Circus Band was directed by the son of one of the residents. Of social interest to the group was the fact that another of the residents formerly played in the band.

Half of the women volunteer group of square dancers dressed in black trousers and white shirts with red bandanas at their throats, as men; their partners were attired in colorful voluminous skirts with colored blouses.

PART PLAYING RHYTHM BAND. A volunteer, formerly a teacher, developed a part-time county home rhythm band or kitchen band which used the instruments as indicated in the rhythm band music, practicing certain musical numbers in part-playing until they were free of mistakes and finally presenting a concert for an activity institute in the Home.

Any activity aide who organized and developed detail in a rhythm band began by asking individually if residents would like to be a part of the band. Two residents were joiners who try anything when asked; some of the others had no other interest and came out of curiosity. Between twelve and sixteen regular members met every Friday afternoon around 2:30 PM in the auditorium.

Instruments were the standard rhythm instruments ordered from a supply company; rhythm sticks are easiest to begin with, just keeping time. The triangle was given to one of the more alert residents to play when that type of sound was needed.

To make rapid progress, it takes a pianist and a band leader, the pianist to play the number through once and then offer suggestions as to what instruments should take different sections of the song. The leader who had to know when each instrument was to play found that pointing a baton at each special player when it was his turn resulted in varying and pleasant sounds.

Players kept their eyes on the leader rather than the pianist so each soloist came in on the correct beat. Confusion resulted when musicians watched the pianist and missed their cue. Practicing for an hour on five or six numbers, the band used the same numbers each week until residents were familiar with their cues.

The afternoon practice ended with two or three old familiar numbers just for fun with residents keeping time in any way they wished. This gave their "brains a rest," as one of them remarked.

The rhythm band program began by using a variety of many kinds of music with definite rhythmic implications, such as march rhythms, waltzes, music for skipping and galloping which have a short-long rhythmic pattern, etc. Music available included some primary music material, some simple piano music, etc. The band members took turns using different instruments, sometimes choosing what they wanted; sometimes the leader determined the instruments to be played. To begin with, the members literally kept time with the instruments they had. Then those with more rhythmic awareness began to experiment with some of the other rhythmic patterns in the music other than the fundamental beat. By using rhythm with variety — some forceful rhythms, some graceful and light, some staccato, the contrasts began to imply the use of different instruments for certain effects such as rhythm sticks for marches and "clocks," etc.; tambourines for Spanish and gypsy music; cymbals for loud chords and emphasis at the end of compositions; a triangle for tinkly effects, and a wood block for hollow sounds.

Rhythm instruments are available in sets, but additional instruments can be added, of course. Many could be homemade: pop-bottle caps, rattles, dowels, rhythm sticks, gourds, etc.

Texts contain rhythm-instrument selections.

SINGO. A pianist, from a list of perhaps thirty songs residents will recognize, prints nineteen on a card resembling a bingo card, with the names of a different song in each square. As with bingo, no two cards should be alike, the arrangement of songs being mixed with a "Free" square in the center.

As the pianist plays part of the song, residents who recognize the tune place a corn kernel or a marker on the card; the first person covering a row in any direction calls "Singo" and may get a prize. Residents usually need a volunteer at the table who can help them see and hear. This can end in a community sing.

To make the cards: make a list of songs for a master copy — as many songs as can be listed which old people are likely to recognize as they're played, such as the following:

> When You and I Were Young Maggie; When Your Hair Has Turned to Silver; My Bonnie; Row, Row, Row Your Boat; Tennessee Waltz; Seeing Nellie Home; Pistol Packing Mama; Indiana; Irene, Good Night; On Wisconsin; Irish Eyes; Beautiful Ohio; For Me and My Gal; Danny Boy; Blue Danube; Five Foot Two; Easter Parade; Jingle Bells; Margie; Dixie; Long Long Trail; Alice Blue Gown; Sailing, Sailing; Isle of Capri; Indian Love Call; Oh, Johnny; Mairzy Doats; Little Brown Jug; Winter Wonderland; Clementine; Blue Skies; You Are My Sunshine; My Blue Heaven; Yankee Doodle; Mary; I've Been Working on the Railroad; Home on the Range; Keep the Home Fires Burning; Roll out the Barrel; America the Beautiful; Love's Old Sweet Song; Santa Claus Is Coming to Town; Swing Low, Sweet Chariot; When I Grow Too Old to Dream; Believe Me, if All Those Endearing Young Charms.

SINGO ☺				
By the Light of the Silvery Moon	I Want a Girl	Let Me Call You Sweetheart	Over There	Dinah
Little Gray Home in the West	My Bonnie	Oh What a Beautiful Morning	Good Old Summer Time	Mary
Bicycle Built for Two	Me and My Gal	Free	Sailing, Sailing	Clementine
Old Oaken Bucket	Mairzy Doates	Take Me out to the Ball Game	I've Been Working on the Railroad	Harvest Moon
Oh Johnny	Keep the Home Fires Burning	Ain't Gonna Rain No More	Long Long Trail	Danny Boy

Fig. 7

Regularly Scheduled Movies

The local theater sends its projectionist to show the county home residents first-run films, and a local group has given the

Home a one thousand dollar screen on which to show the movies.

Evening movies are best shown in the winter in rooms where windows cannot ordinarily be completely covered. Unless a room is totally darkened, afternoon movies can't be seen. Sometimes a 16mm movie can be shown down a hall lined with chairs and the adjoining doors closed. Movie shorts of animals and children, local, old-fashioned or familiar settings, colored or scenic, unsophisticated, sentimental and sweet movies seem most popular. Since TV is also a type of spectator activity, movie shorts of other varieties than those shown of TV should be selected.

Some of the most popular movies or slides are shown by amateur camera clubs or by traveled volunteers; even seeing unspectacular, local Home movies are happy experiences both because the residents know the photographer and commentator and because they recognize or are interested in the setting. But the great value is the pleasure of joining a small group seated together who can interrupt to ask questions in folksy, informal chat. In one of the Homes, a local camera club can be depended upon to come in Tuesday evenings to bring together a group of residents in entertainment and friendship.

A staff member says, "Our residents go to bed at 6:30 PM," but finds that if there is an early evening activity to stay up for, they will stay up. Certainly, nurses don't want residents to go to bed at 6:30 PM knowing they'll never stay in bed twelve hours.

A volunteer or resident may run the projector so that movies can be held more frequently; free movies are available locally or from a number of free film sources.

To take a movie marquee, one uses a large cardboard box, cutting off one side and attaching the box to the side of a post in the hall and placing a string of Christmas tree lights around the edge of the box; the box is decorated with crepe paper and is notched, and the name of the movie on a strip of paper is inserted along the sides; the box is exhibited and lighted the day of the movie.

News Media

Home Newspaper Reporters' Press Club

Home newspapers are rexographed and mimeographed in the

Home or arrangements are made to have this done outside the Home. Residents often meet weekly to plan and assign news stories and feature interviews; staff meetings help unite the group in covering the news, giving assignments, submitting copy and discussing news ideas.

To get names in the paper, reporters often list visitors or residents who make trips outside the Home, attend activities in the Home for the first time or are responsible for special accomplishments. Any justified recognition is important. The Home newspaper reporter publicizes the monthy activity schedule and prints regularly appearing columns; announces employee changes; acknowledges staff or volunteers; lists donations and prize winners; writes columns: Lost and Found, Wanted or For Sale; writes book reports; does a column on people with special jobs in the Home; writes a movie review; does a name scramble; has a poetry corner; reports on sports, listing tournament winners; presents conundrums, contests and written quizzes; has a continued story; writes obituaries and short biographies; lists new residents and personnel; gives monthly birthdays; announces church services and volunteer schedules and vacations.

Home Newsletter Excerpts

Let's Get Acquainted

(By a New Activity Aide)

There may be a lot of people in our Home whom you haven't met here but with whom you have grown up. I hope that each month we can introduce a few of you, and if you find anything in common with someone you read about—look him up.

Since I'm anxious to get better acquainted with all of you, I'm going to set aside every Tuesday and Thursday morning from 9:00 to 10:00 to visit you. Maybe you'll tell me about yourselves or we could just talk. I've started on the second floor, Room 200, and plan to work right down to the ground floor. I think you'll know where I've been; and if you'd rather not participate, just say so;

but I would appreciate a welcome and I'll look forward to meeting you. If I should miss you, look me up in the activity room on the ground floor.

My first visits were in the following rooms:

.... is rather new here and making herself at home. She is one of my cheerful, willing right hands. Chances are it won't take long to get to know her and enjoy her as I do. Room 202: Mr. and Mrs. ...., are a very charming husband and wife who lived in Waterman forty years before coming to the Home. Until retirement, he was a maintenance engineer at the Pet® Milk Dairy. Their son-in-law . . .

Our Home News which is now in its fourth year of publication continues to be popular and much appreciated. It is something every Home should have—mostly as a reminder of records—services, birthdays, new residents and tributes to those who have passed away—important features. Poems or articles written by patients—jokes or fillers found in magazines handed to the editor because of some special appeal—that is all it takes, and you have your own publication . . .

Editor of the **Madison Capital Times** invited all the residents to a lutefisk supper. He assured us this would be an annual event—it was fun preparing for it—decorating the dining room, planning Norwegian garb for all the girls who helped to prepare or serve the food—watching the smirks and smiles of our Norwegians, and the looks of skeptic surprise on the faces of those who had never eaten lutefisk—**and didn't** like it.

Your Home newsletter correspondent is one of the residents, a victim of multiple sclerosis, confined to a wheelchair, but blessed with hands, eyes and mind fairly intact and so takes an active interest in life at the Home. She also writes weekly columns for two local newspapers.

One Home newspaper included want ads. Wanted: 500 players, poker player. Wanted: Contributors of news items for the **Pulse**—residents, staff or volunteers. Found: a poet among our residents
....

A new column appearing in the Home paper is called the "Trading Post" to help residents who would like to buy a particular item or would like to sell an article they no longer can use. There will be no charge for the listing of items. All you need do is contact .... on third floor, East Room 361, and he will take your ad. It will then appear in the **County Home Reporter's** next issue. You deal with the person directly. The employees may also have items listed. Should you have houses, cows, or kittens for sale, list them and expect results. We have a circulation of about 300, so let's go and get the economy moving forward.

The first advertiser on our list is a man who has two transistor radios which he would like to trade for one radio that will work in the basement so that he can enjoy the ball games. See .... in the commissary.

For sale: one pair of pillow cases and three luncheon cloths. See .... has for sale a new necktie and a pair of overshoes, size seven. .... has a Timex wrist watch for sale at a reasonable price, in good running order. .... has daily and Sunday **Milwaukee Journals** for sale. See him for delivery service.

Residents are interested in the teenage volunteers' names and schools listed in their Home newspaper.

In a column headed "Spotlights on ....," the oldest resident on down to the youngest is featured, one each issue.

The **Home News** sponsors a contest:

The prize will not be paid more than once to any one contestant within a year's time. However, honorable mention will

> be given those with the largest lists, if
> they have won before; and at the end of
> the calendar year a special prize will be
> paid to the contestant who has topped the
> list most often. Get as many three letter
> words as you can in the words . . . .
> (Fourth of July, August Picnic, County
> Fair or Summer Vacation, etc.).

The Infirmary Tatler has a column, "Nursing Service," which includes lists of residents who have "shown marked improvement," "He attempts to feed himself and to stand with help," etc.

A Home newsheet announced that all reporters will receive notebooks with their names imprinted on the front cover, a help in keeping notes on the meetings and making reports. At each meeting the staff of residents discusses the article they found to be the most interesting in the previous issue and gives the reasons why.

The Tatler has several interesting pages of resident interviews on some timely national news, such as interviews on the orbital flights — outstanding impressions of the flight, how space flights will affect world military situations, "should we or should we not share our space knowledge?" and other comments from sixteen residents interviewed.

A Home recently announced the winner of a contest to name the newly published Home newspaper at a dance for hospital patients and residents.

The Tatler has a column headed "Plaque of Honor, Deep Appreciation, Three Cheers."

> Too often we do not take time out from
> our busy schedule to give "thank you's"
> when they are due. We'd like to say a
> special "thank you" to one who has given
> of herself and her time to us over a period
> of many years full measure (and it de-
> scribes the volunteer, her attitude, her
> assignments in the Home and her hours
> of work.)

A new column, "Who Is She?" is included in the paper:

> She works on the new press every day,
> pressing men's pants and the dentist's
> jacket. She should be praised for the good

> job that she does. She works on the **Chip-Co-Life** and studies French. She likes to be alone. How could she study if she didn't like to be alone? Who is she?

A newspaper, **Out Our Way**, is typed in caps which are more easily read.

Stapling and distributing the news sheet can be important jobs for residents in wheelchairs, saving employees' time.

> We, the Press Club, have completed one full year of putting together the monthly paper, the **County Home Reporter.** Our mailing list has grown to fifty-eight paid subscriptions and eighteen free copies which are mailed to other Homes like ours in the state. One subscription goes to Switzerland and another to Hawaii. Approximately 200 copies are distributed to residents and employees here in the Home.

Writing for the Local Paper

These are items that could be reported:

1. Visit of the district physical therapist, state personnel visitors.
2. Announcement of the completed enclosed runway for ambulatory and wheelchair patients.
3. Acknowledgment of a letter and gift of money for the activity fund in memory of a deceased friend.
4. Looking back a year ago, three years, five years to admissions and deaths in the Home that month.
5. Announcement and review of the films shown.
6. Visitors who took the resident for a ride, describing the trip and friends whom they visited.
7. Announcement of church services, musical selections, pianist, notes on the sermon.
8. Lists of visitors and their locale.
9. Birthday party, celebrants and gifts presented by the residents in the Home.
10. Visits of the infirmary trustees.

11. Descriptions of holiday and seasonal decorations in the Home.

12. Announcements of changes in staff, births, anniversaries and trips.

13. Announcing transfers of residents to other hospitals for surgery or further care.

14. Lists of prize winners at the parties, list of residents who are being introduced to new hobbies.

15. Announcement of rummage sales in the Home, open-house affairs, etc.

16. Listing leisure time activities, as well as regularly scheduled activities.

17. Congratulations to grandfathers and great grandfathers with new grandchildren.

18. Announcement of craft exhibits or craft sales.

19. Original poems.

20. Listing blood donors from the Home.

21. Listing names and addresses from admiring and distant readers.

22. The arrival of the first pussy-willows in the Home, receiving the bouquet used at the visiting senator's banquet in town, arrival of the first robin, effects of being snowbound in the Home.

23. Easter-bonnet parade and other holiday festivities.

24. Special requests. (Chicken necks, a favorite of the group, were ordered; the activity aide cooked them till they were well done and seasoned them. They ate these with pickles, onion Saltine® crackers and soda pop! — a menu they chose.)

Radio Broadcasts

On a Home radio broadcasting system rigged up by the superintendent, the activity aide reads aloud from the Home newspaper as well as the local papers; residents listen to favorite or familiar music on records or tapes, hold interviews or contests and play games.

A local radio station had a series of interviews with more able and more easily interviewed residents which has stimulated radio listening in the Home.

A singing group of residents found to their surprise that the man from the radio station, who was present at the back of the room, had been making a tape recording which he played back to them and which he later played on the radio program. The Poetry Reading Club invited him to make tape recordings at their meetings.

Since a resident sent a rug he had made to a radio program called Party Line, the crafts in the Home are mentioned every week on the radio. The radio announcer who called the Home while on the air to inquire how the listeners could be of help has recruited two beauticians through the announcement.

Choral Reading

In the era in which residents lived they enjoyed reading aloud together during happy evenings at home with their families as children or as young adults. Choral reading, which nicely adapts this old skill, can accommodate a group which can see to read. No other special talent is necessary — everyone takes part on an equal basis, finding self expression and special recognition in being given a "part to do."

Steps

1. From a book in the library the leader decides on a simple poem with choral reading directions. The poetry selections may be typed in capital letters and mimeographed to be distributed and read more easily.

2. He selects a place and time when residents are already assembled and the light is suitable for reading.

3. He reads the selection aloud for the readers perhaps asking them about the mood and meanings as they understand them.

4. He assigns part-reading to residents who like to do it; residents may decide who should do the solos. Divisions and groups are taken by whatever grouping seems natural, perhaps as they happen to sit, in groups or rows or part of the circle. Choice of special parts should never be limited to talents but rather to

those residents who may be most benefited by it; and as the group continues, the importance of these ego-builders may be seen.

Assigned Parts[2]

Leader: The person in charge.

Solo: Anyone selected, a different person for each; solo 1, 2, 3 and so on. A solo could mean that this person may have a chance to be recognized in this way, something that is often important to him.

Duet: Two residents reading together.

Groups: 1, 2, 3 and 4 are used for variety of words or phrases.

Division: The group taking part is divided into two equal sections, probably with some line of demarcation, perhaps around the circle, men or women, etc.

All: Everyone speaking together.

Residents may help select poems from newspapers or magazines, poems they have memorized as children or will select from books of poetry and indicating reading parts which are most effective. They can suggest the pauses in the lines and the spacing between words. The leader may count, either silently or aloud, "one, two" or tap his foot two counts until the group gets the feeling of the rhythm.

Any jingle in four-four time is easy and fun.

Poetry that is excellent for choral reading by oldsters can be found in **Choral Readings for Fun and Recreation,** edited by Harry J. Heltman and Helen A. Brown and published by the Westminster Press in Philadelphia. Two more books, **Choral Readings from the Bible** and **Choral Readings for Fun and Inspiration** contain good material too. They are also published by Westminster Press.

---

[2] Reprinted from **Choral Readings for Fun and Recreation,** ed. Helen A. Brown and Harry J. Heltman. Copyright 1956, W. L. Jenkins. The Westminster Press. Used by permission.

Bible Class

Occasionally, transportation is arranged by volunteers for residents attending a local church. Hopefully the Home chaplains or pastoral visitors will study the aged and infirm to determine suitable satisfaction of spiritual needs. Every effort should be made to see that residents are not separated from the community church if they are able to attend services there.

Besides the religious services conducted by local lay people, ministers or priests, good use is made of radio, TV and recordings in bringing religion to the Homes.

If requested, congregations will make services available as well as distribute educational pamphlets and church bulletins to all residents, whether or not they are church members.

The goals of these religious activities should be to help the aged find "opportunities for greatness." One should remember the quote, "The test of a people is how it behaves toward the old."

Through fellowship and faith, the aged meet problems of advanced years with more tranquility and less fear, finding strengthened resources in their religion.

In a time of life often characterized by sickness, tribulation, and regression, religion brings hope for the resident's tomorrow. Those who care for the aged are concerned with uniting broad efforts toward seeing that each resident receives the benefits, both spiritual and material, that he needs.

Nonsectarian Homes sometimes hesitate to conduct Bible classes because of the threat of disagreement, but many successful and regularly scheduled classes are in progress. Church services, sometimes possible with a portable altar in the bed patient's room, are conducted weekly or several times a week. In one Home, a tape recording is made of the city church services and played the following Friday in the Home.

A local minister or dependable lay person, in one nursing home a retired minister, comes weekly to join the residents in singing hymns together, reading the Bible, seeing Biblical slides, studying a Sunday school lesson and answering Biblical quizzes as a nonsectarian group. In one Home a "project for missions" means knitting or sewing something requested by a foreign mission; interestingly, the missionaries send slides back to the nursing home showing the people in foreign countries receiving the gifts, which gives the project special value.

Meeting weekly with a volunteer, residents have made a scrapbook of religious articles which are used to substitute religious services which may be cancelled. The articles may be read by a resident or staff person without special preparation.

A resident who enrolled in a Bible course from a state extension division finds this study worthwhile and interesting.

"We sang Thanksgiving hymns from mimeographed sheets, then we all joined in the hymn, 'Count Your Blessings,' after which each person was asked to name his own personal blessings. Many were astonished at the countless ones they could enumerate which they had never considered as such," a resident says.

A Resident Council

Residents are selected who show the greatest aptitude and interest in recreational activities and they are asked to become council members to help plan and run the program. The council should not be too large but should be representative of the residents in the Home.

Functions of a council could be as follows:

1. To give the residents a voice in planning the programs.
2. To promote interest among other residents.
3. To recruit residents' opinions and reactions to the program.
4. To strengthen the feeling of belonging.
5. To create and develop recreational ideas of its own.
6. To advertise and promote the program within the Home.

Council meetings should be held regularly, subcommittees formed and minutes kept.

A resident council assigns members to "adopt" new residents as they're admitted to the Home in an attempt to prevent these people being lonely or feeling lost. Fourteen residents meet weekly to discuss program planning, gather news for the Home newspaper, serve on helpful committees reaching the hard to reach and doing more for themselves and more for others.

After organizing a residents' council, an occupational therapist serving as leader of the council at first found residents extremely hesitant about making suggestions for bettering their life in the Home, since they thought of suggestions as complaints which they felt they shouldn't indulge in, as they were afraid of some unknown form of reprimand.

In organizing the council, a list of potential council members made up by the nurses and occupational therapist was mimeographed, a copy of which was sent to each council member recruit: "You have been appointed by the staff to attend the resident council meeting in occupational therapy at 9:30 AM every Wednesday morning. We are looking forward to these meetings from which we hope will grow a better Home for all our residents."

So little response followed this that it was necessary for the leaders to go up on the wards and insist that the residents come, although in time they all came voluntarily and waited for the others. Some of them who wouldn't say a word soon made many worthwhile suggestions when they were told all their ideas couldn't be used but could be discussed. "Now the council members are so officious, they are jealous of giving up their position," the therapist says.

Suggesting several times that other residents could take over for them or share with them on the council, the leaders found them not yet ready to accept other residents as members; in fact, they asked other residents to leave when they came to the door. Nor have they expressed a desire to have a president or secretary; the leaders are waiting for them to want and accept others. When the council began to ask personnel to the meeting, inviting attendants, cooks and the doctor, the leaders knew that the residents were growing and developing as a council unit.

Starting with the hope that in some small way they could create a feeling of cohesiveness among the members, the leaders helped them direct their thinking into a more positive channel, to create interest in working towards a better Home through their participation, an ego strengthener which would spread to other residents. Residents often lose direction and purpose, become hypercritical and find themselves competing, but the council has noticed some growth and has activated many members.

Direction toward more projects gives residents prestige in doing work for someone else, a realistic activity which gives a large amount of gratification. A solution to the question of how to get the residents started has been in directing responsibility to them, and the results have been rewarding.

Although the council isn't told, this is in essence group therapy, discussing their problems and learning how to deal with them.

In another Home the residents have drawn up their own bylaws:

Bylaws of a Residents' Committee (Residents' Council)

Name

The group shall be known as the "Residents' Committee."

Purpose

1. To provide an opportunity for regular discussion of matters of interest to the residents of the Home.
2. To promote friendship and foster charity among the residents.
3. To provide a channel of communication between management and residents in order to promote greater understanding and cooperation.

    A. Aid, assist and inform management regarding resident desires, etc., in the area of recreation, craft and entertainment.

Officers

1. The officers of the committee shall be president, vice president, secretary, and treasurer.
2. The Board of Directors shall consist of the superintendent and two assistants, one to act as moderator.

Meetings

Meetings shall take place at the time and place chosen by the officers and approved by the superintendent.

Duties of Officers

1. The term of office shall begin at the adjournment of the meeting at which they were elected.
2. The president shall preside at all meetings and in his absence, the vice president presides.
3. The secretary shall keep accurate minutes of the meetings, one copy to go to the board of directors.
4. The treasurer shall report quarterly the financial position of the residents' recreation fund.

Finding Work in the Home

Older and disabled members may make productive and useful contributions to the community in which they live, depending on their abilities. One important job is the stamping of medical forms for medical services; over 336,000 envelopes were stuffed for the Easter Seal Society, the Lions Club, cancer fund or other crusade agencies. Fund drives for retarded children and cerebral palsy are on the list as well as the Red Cross at Christmas each year.

Everyone "benefits directly or indirectly from these activities; the physically handicapped are amazed to find a need for their services long after they have been convinced their usefulness to society is over."

One resident keeps busy rolling bandages, a never-ending job, because these "wraps" are washed over and over again and then must be wound. Another operates the addressograph machine and is proud of being useful. Others grind sharp points on the small American flags to be used Memorial Day, or they operate the splicing machine.

The sewing room is supervised by an employee where residents are busy mending sheets and underwear, making aprons and tie-strings for gowns and aprons, snipping foam rubber for stuffing cushions for wheelchairs.

Capable residents who want to be useful assume responsibility for feeding others unable to feed themselves. If they understand their role, they are dependable and efficient and aware of their part in the routine of the Home.

They can themselves be benefited by being useful in small ways. For nursing-care-patients in the Home, residents make large bibs from bolts of toweling: turn up the bottom edge to catch the crumbs, turn down the top to absorb spilling, and cut out and bind a curved neck.

The oldster usually likes familiar work — mowing the lawn, raking the leaves, working at the switchboard (work he's done before), working in the stockroom delivering supplies in various parts of the Home, working in the Home kitchen, dining room or tidying up areas. He is busy, helpful and much happier.

Responsible residents take commissary carts to the ward selling supplies of tobacco, Kleenex®, lotion, candy and comfort articles. People who can be responsible for keys, making change and ordering supplies, can keep a cart stocked and in good service. In one Home with ambulatory residents only, the commissary is in charge of residents who also sell craft items made by residents, and coffee and snacks at cost made in the Home cooking class. Some of the Homes accept clean used clothing, as well as jewelry and "white elephants" donated by the volunteers; residents set a price and sell the items to one another for a few cents, building up the "activity fund."

Residents sometimes prefer paying for donated clothing and want the self-respect of going to the "store" in the Home, trying on the garment for size, style and color and paying a few cents for it.

A retired librarian, now in a wheelchair, catalogues the books and assumes the responsibilities of a professional librarian. The library is open, and she is there several hours every day.

One helps him to retain as much of his independence as possible ... A goal for each day: to introduce some new job idea to a resident.

Are there residents who can do the following?

1. Serve at a reception desk? Work in the kitchen?

2. Deliver the newspapers?

3. Collect meal tickets at the dining room door?

4. Refinish old furniture in the storeroom?

Any resident able to enjoys taking a book cart (which could be a discarded medicine cart) to the wards. Current unclaimed magazines may be picked up at any post office on a regular basis.

The Home newspaper says:

Where in the wide world are there finer people than the men and women who live in our Home! Just let the word go out that there is rhubarb, beans, or asparagus to prepare for freezing, and we almost have more people offer to help than we have knives! And it's such fun when we all put our aprons on and sit around the long counter, laugh together and even have a cup of coffee when the work is finished. That's when we know the meaning of our Home.

It's each of us helping in one way or another — like .... keeping all our knives sharp, like .... who used to keep all our flower beds such a thing of beauty, like .... helping the cook, (lists the others) who three times a day do dishes and set the table.

One of our men repairs TV's and radios in the basement area. Another, having brought his tools and equipment, repairs and re-upholsters furniture for the Home. Another shells hickory nuts, walnuts and butternuts to sell for one dollar a pound.

Our residents painted the curbs outside the Home when the street was new. Four of our men painted the lawn benches and the lawn furniture in the spring.

One of our residents repairs electric equipment, does wood working jobs for the Home, another gives haircuts and repairs shoes.

Chapter XII

ACTIVITIES FOR RESIDENTS WITH SOME USE OF THEIR HANDS

A merry heart doeth good like medicine, but a broken spirit drieth up the bones. Proverbs XVII V. 2.

COOKING CLASSES

Cooking is a "natural" for most women and occasionally for men residents too; if the schedules and facilities in the Home kitchen permit, approval may be given for using the kitchen an hour or two during midafternoon for a cooking class. Residents in one Home have a weekly morning class, six women in wheelchairs making bread or applekuchen, brownies or cookies. During the pre-Christmas season they package fancy Christmas pastry and fruit cake and sell it. In a snack bar operated by residents and opened every afternoon and evening, the food made in the cooking class is served with coffee and sold at cost to residents who enjoy inviting a visitor for a treat while they chat.

Facilities for cooking have been built in a craft shop — cupboards, refrigerator, stove, and tables; or a workable kitchen no longer used for preparing meals is used by a residents' cooking class. Because they have difficulty in seeing, residents use a large recipe sign set up with two-inch-high letters posted on the table. Forgetful residents always need a great deal of supervision so that the recipe is closely followed. Quick mixes are easy if cooking facilities are limited, but residents usually prefer the old familiar recipes which they know by heart.

In one cooking class, residents also discuss correct table settings. In other Homes, the activity aides have taken residents into their own homes on a weekly basis, making cookies and so on.

A cooking class had a cooking demonstration from a power and light company making Christmas breads and a local florist gave them a flower-arranging demonstration for a second afternoon feature. In another Home, the gas and electric company demonstrated "New Trends in Home Making" with new appliances, saucepans, cleansing agents, packaged foods, starches and other household helps, previous to a discussion in which they could take part.

A Home cooking class sold baked goods to employees and bought mixers, mixing bowls and pans and decided one week what they wanted to do the next week. At an ice cream social each man dressed up and invited a lady friend and the cooking class baked eleven rhubarb pies which were served in the get-together. Sometimes the aide posts a sign inviting anyone who'd like to cook; other times she goes on the wards and announces "Who's ready for the cooking class?"

Recipes for the Cooking Class without a Stove
Butterscotch Toffee Delight

1½ cup whipping cream
1 can (5½ oz) butterscotch syrup (topping)
½ teaspoon vanilla extract
1 unfrosted angel cake (9½")

¾ pound English toffee, crushed (put through food grinder using largest blade)

Whip cream until it starts to thicken. Add butterscotch syrup and vanilla slowly and continue beating until thick. Cut cake into three layers — horizontally. Spread the butterscotch mixture on the layers and sprinkle each generously with crushed toffee.

Put cake back together again and frost the top and sides with butterscotch mixture and sprinkle them, too, with toffee. Place cake in the refrigerator and chill for a minimum of six hours. Serves twelve.

Bremerton Balls
No-cook rum cookies!

2½ cups crushed vanilla wafers (most of a 12-oz pkg.)
2 tablespoons cocoa
1 cup confectioner's sugar (sift before measuring)

1 cup chopped walnuts
3 tablespoons corn syrup or honey
1 tablespoon rum extract
confectioner's sugar for topping

Mix well the crumbs, cocoa, the one cup sugar and the nuts. Add the corn syrup and extract. Mix all very thoroughly.

Form into inch size balls, then roll in confectioners' sugar. Keep in covered tin. Makes three to three and a half dozen cookies. These are even better the second day.

Recipes for the Cooking Class with a Stove

Spiced Raisin Cookies

1 cup water	1 teaspoon baking powder
2 cups raisins	1 teaspoon baking soda
1 cup shortening	1 teaspoon salt
2 cups sugar	¼ teaspoon allspice
3 eggs	1½ teaspoon cinnamon
1 teaspoon vanilla extract	¼ teaspoon nutmeg
4 cups flour	

Boil the water and raisins together for five minutes and set aside to cool. Cream shortening and sugar well. Add eggs to the creamed mixture and beat well. Add the vanilla to the raisin mixture. Sift the dry ingredients together and add to the creamed mixture and mix well. Add the cooled raisin and water mixture and blend. Drop by teaspoon onto greased cookie sheet. Bake for twelve minutes at 350° F.

Goblin's Cider

1 quart sweet apple cider	½ cup brown sugar
8 whole allspice	few grains of salt
8 whole cloves	1 stick cinnamon

Put cider into saucepan, add spices, and sugar; cover and heat very slowly to boiling. Heat should be so low that it takes the cider half an hour to come to a boil. Remove from heat and strain. Serves five.

Poppy Seed Cake

½ cup poppy seed	1 teaspoon vanilla extract
½ cup evaporated milk	⅛ teaspoon salt
½ cup water	2 cups sifted flour
½ cup shortening	2 teaspoons baking powder
1½ cups sugar	4 egg whites

Mix milk and water, add to poppy seed and let stand one hour. Cream shortening. Add sugar and vanilla, and cream until light and fluffy. Add poppy seed and milk. Mix, then add sifted dry ingredients. Fold in egg whites which have been beaten stiff, but not dry. Pour into two well-greased 9″ layer cake pans. Bake in moderate oven (350° F.) until a toothpick inserted in the center comes out clean, about 30 to 35 minutes. Let layers cool in pan about five minutes, then turn out on racks to finish cooling. When cold, frost with mint icing.

Frosted Baked Apples

½ cup sugar	melted butter
1 cup water	sugar
6 baking apples	shredded coconut

Boil the sugar and the water together for two minutes. Core the apples and pare the upper halves. Roll each apple in the melted butter, then in sugar.

TYPING

A typing book from a secondhand store and a secondhand typewriter may make this skill possible. A spastic with no use of his hands types with his head — a stick at his forehead attached to a band around his head; a blind man types his poetry for the Home newspaper. If residents are proficient enough, they may type letters for those unable to write.

CRAFTS

Recreation programs often start with crafts, partly because the activity aide feels most secure in this area and because a craft is a tangible thing, something to be seen, admired and used. To produce and to achieve are drives that lie close to the core of everyone and persist as long as life itself, although often they are buried far beneath the surface. Combining work with the hands and the mental concentration necessary to create something makes for growth. What the oldster has in his hands exists because he made it; rehabilitation is hastened or he's assisted in the adjustment to his disability.

It is felt that crafts are usually only a small part of the program since many times they reach only a small percentage of the residents: those people who can see well enough or use their hands well enough to make a craft. One must find a use and a need for the craft: Can it be sold, given as a gift, used in the

Home or community? No one is willing to spend time in useless "busy-work," and suggesting such a thing is an insult to an adult of any age! Too often the craft made in the Home is one which the activity aide likes, his selection, his idea of what would be fun to do. If the resident can see the craft, he knows whether or not he wants to make it; and if he's told how it's going to be used, he will decide whether or not he wants to make the effort.

Women residents who do handiwork are busy with their own wardrobes, usually enjoy taking care of their rooms and socialize more easily than men. The hands of aged men sometimes lack strength to do heavy carpentry work or any fine work; and because motivation with them is often especially difficult, this book stresses crafts for men.

Disposing of Crafts

MAKING PRIZES. How to dispose of the things made in the craft shop! One Home makes all their own bingo prizes as an incentive in promoting craft work in the shop. The prize should be something of little monetary value, but something which can be used — repaired jewelry, a decorated fly swatter, a decorated waste-paper basket, a tin can covered with cord to be used for a vase or a pencil holder, a decorated handkerchief, a clamp ash tray for a wheelchair, scuffs, a boutonniere, a decorated pencil and pad or a fancy party hat, etc.

DISPLAYING AN EXHIBIT (at the county fair, community fall festival, or local church bazaar). Most of the county fairs have exhibits submitted by county home residents who get blue ribbons for rugs, quilts or aprons.

A Home is planning an annual booth at the county fair through which they hope to acquaint the community with activities carried on in the Home. Every thing displayed will be made by the resident: cutting boards, cork coasters, serving trays and hot pads, flowers grown in the garden, crocheted and knitted items and dolls in many colors.

CRAFT SALES. Residents at an annual Christmas sale (preparations having been made for months), sold mosaic tile hot stands, pillow cases, dresser scarves, table cloths, toaster covers, shopping bags, dish towels, pot holders, stuffed animals, mittens, bed slippers, handkerchiefs, rugs, pin-cushions, hockey caps, pajama bags, clown dolls, doll cradles, magazine racks, yard ornaments, rocking ducks, bird feeder trays, cigarette holders and knife holders, foot stools, lawn chairs, rocker hobby horses, hanging book shelves, doll furniture, flower stands, weather vanes, picnic trays, wall plaques, whatnot shelves, bird houses, tie racks, copper enameling, textile painting, scrapbooks, purses and flower vases.

Approximately 500 people attended the sale, over 300 of whom signed for the mailing list, relatives and employees not included, with about $600.00 taken in from purchases. Volunteers were kept busy wrapping packages. Residents had a part in making articles for the sale, working in an assembly line fashion, one man doing the sanding, another, the painting, etc., so that specific articles were not assigned to individuals.

PROJECTS FOR THE COMMUNITY. Residents help the community by folding bandages for the Red Cross or cancer societies, making scrapbooks for orphanages, rattles for pediatric wards at the local hospital or quilts for families whose homes have been wiped out by fire.

For many of the elderly who have spent their lives busily working at a job, the best form of recreation is productive work. Homemaking programs for teenage girls could be developed by the presence and advice of older women who have won blue ribbons at local fairs or who learned to cook on a wood-burning stove. Old fishermen can teach junior seamen; old farmers are useful in 4H programs and old tinsmiths can teach their craft to teenagers.

A resident who knits mittens for "all the nurses" formerly taught children knitting who came to visit the Home. Of Norwegian birth, he learned knitting as a child himself.

In another Home, residents work long hours every day making layettes for needy babies and clothes for children up to twelve years of age; new material as well as eight sewing machines have been donated by the county Homemakers and senior citizen groups for residents working on the projects.

Says one aide:

You can feel a difference in their attitude in being in the Home and being useful to the community through this project; they've found someone who needs them. Residents who have only "taken in" on the receiving end as long as I've been here, are now giving.

They're here before I open the doors in the morning and stay on after I'm supposed to have left at night. Before this, they had little chance to show appreciation toward anyone; they only received and so had become selfish. This sewing project for the needy children has put them on the "giving end" of life.

We began by talking with the social worker about Christmas presents for children; material for clothes and layettes have been given, and money donated for materials and for items residents can't make, like boys' clothes.

A gift package for a new baby made by residents in the Home includes two drawstring nighties, two dozen diapers, two blankets with crocheted edges, bibs, a stuffed animal, pins and two sacques (summer and winter baby jackets). These items are put in plastic bags when complete and put in a box to be picked up by someone from the welfare department. Over sixty boxes with complete sets of these items have been made, assembled and given to the welfare office this summer.

The residents enjoy the project by working together on it — some sew on the sewing machine, some do hand-work on the hems, sort buttons, feather stitch or crochet, some of which they take to their rooms; others are able to cut out patterns, press or do some of the other details of preparation. One granddaughter works as a volunteer cutting patterns.

Men make miniature furniture, for which women make the mattresses, pillows and bed clothing, as well as the stuffed dolls and animals.

"Since children's clothing and baby layettes are so expensive, this is one of the nicest services we can think of," a representative of the county welfare department says. "The recipients are all children with no father, or a deserting father. Some of the recipients are not eligible for public assistance. Many of the children have never had anything new; the things they've always worn have been hand-me-downs. Now the older children say, 'We won't put this new clothing on the baby until the baby has been bathed'; so it is teaching children good baby hygiene and good grooming for themselves."

Reading to children in a story hour, a resident helps on a community project at the public library thus delighting the children and giving the mothers a helping hand and enjoyment to himself.

In May, residents count poppies for the annual American Legion Auxiliary Poppy Day, thus serving the community. In another Home, given the materials and directions, residents make plastic wreaths to be placed on veterans' graves.

Residents' scrapbooks serve a dual purpose by "bringing pleasure to those who make them, as well as those who look at them"; one of the residents makes books of religious pictures from old calendars.

Over 900 dressings were once folded in three and a half hours by twenty residents for Oshkosh VNA. A letter from VNA on the bulletin board read:

> To the Busy Beavers: As you made up the cancer dressings, you may have considered it only a project. To the many sick people who will be using these dressings, you are a hovering angel. It is a help to the Visiting Nurse Association to have these dressings all assembled, wrapped and ready to go when the need arises. Please know your time and labor is appreciated. God bless you all.

The doctor, a Shriner who has made a hobby of clowning at children's orphanages and benefits for crippled children, has set a theme for the oldsters in the Home who made and sold dozens of clown dolls in their craft shop.

A resident writes:

> What fun it is to make a "Yo-Yo" clown doll! I have made them, and children's eyes brightened when they saw them. Calico circles 2″ in diameter are pressed and cut. Circles are seamed at the edges, gathered into discs, then strung together with heavy cord to form the body. The heads are made of white fabric. The eyes, nose, and mouth may be painted or embroidered on the face; a clown cap is sewed to the head and a gay ruffle placed around the neck. One can use originality in finishing the dolls and could even make a "Yo-Yo" having a rabbit's head for Easter.

Making quilts for underprivileged children or needy families, one of the Homes made forty crib-sized quilts given underprivileged children and five full-sized quilts were presented to needy families in the community. A great deal of pride goes into these labors of love, every stitch being done by hand in a weekly afternoon project directed by Red Cross. The city department stores, as well as the volunteers, supply the new scrap materials and remnants.

In another Home, volunteers distribute the materials, each women resident completing a block in two week's time when the volunteers return with a quilting frame, the batting and the material for the underside of the quilt. Men in the Home say, "We used to do this for our wives," and tie the quilt and complete it in an afternoon's time. The Home, in this way, produces a quilt every two weeks. In another Home, a quilt made by residents was raffled off, $48.00 worth of chances being sold to employees in the Home for the "activity fund."

Made especially high for wheelchairs, quilting frames in the Home craft room accommodate three residents sitting there together tying a comforter a day for anyone who brings them the materials.

Residents, after completing a quilt which was sent to earthquake victims at Anchorage, Alaska, were excited when they received the following letter:

Mrs. E. S. Wales
Executive Secretary
Randolph Chapter
American Red Cross
Randolph, Wisconsin

Dear Mrs. Wales:

The two very attractive patchwork quilts brought great joy to one of our disaster sufferers.

You might inform the kind donors that the quilts were given to a single man, age 74, who lives alone and suffered the complete loss of his home and furnishings. He is supported by Social Security and a small retirement check.

The Red Cross purchased a furnished trailer for this man, and the quilts afforded color and warmth.

*He was delighted, and sends his warmest greetings and
deepest thanks to all who worked on the quilts.*

Sincerely,
Miss Margaret Stanning
Casework Supervisor

Stuffing animals and dolls for children in the community
as community projects give residents special incentive. One
inquires first of community welfare groups as to the need, the
kind of project requested, and the number of items which could
be used. Adopting children in orphanages, helping children receiving public welfare assistance or helping needy families referred
by churches may suggest possible projects for a year round work
class scheduled for a definite time, perhaps once or twice a week.
Although residents will want to work individually on projects
during evenings and week-ends, meeting regularly will help
remind them of goals and will help to structure a unified and
dedicated group.

Scraps of material with a pattern for stuffed animals and dolls
from the dime store and a supply of old donated nylon stockings,
may be the incentive necessary for the lady residents joining the
Sunset Suzies or Sewing Sisters. A cup of coffee or a mint to
pass, some fruit or a cookie, a chairman and a committee and
they are incorporated. Perhaps the piece-work system can be
best used, one person cutting from the pattern, one sewing on
the sewing machine or by hand and those still more infirm cutting
up nylon stockings preparatory to stuffing. But the "cause" must
be important: "To be needed, to be useful, to help someone
underprivileged."

Dear Friends at Sunny Ledge:

*We wish to acknowledge receipt of your donations of
stuffed dolls. These story book dolls and character dolls are
very unusual indeed, and our youngsters have been fascinated
with them. On behalf of our children we extend to each of
the ladies who have a part in making this unusual donation
possible, our most sincere thanks and appreciation.*

Sincerely,
Administrator
Shriners Hospital for Crippled Children

Reviving Interest in Old Familiar Craft Activities

A resident wanted the Home to bring him the equipment from the jewelry shop where he worked for thirty years before he had a stroke and came to the Home to live. There were two possibilities in basement areas for his working on this old familiar craft; the aide thought of using a chicken wire frame around his table where he worked on watches and clocks and where the watch bands he displayed for sale would be protected. Finally he chose the area he liked best. The staff was amazed that he could sit on a stool, working with the infirmities of his stroke, amazed at his determination in returning to a skill he loved.

A ninety-year-old still over six feet tall who reads palms and is also interested in analyzing hand writing, finds this an easy way to make friends since everyone is interested in what someone else has to say about him; he makes "good use of the hands" of others in reviving an old interest.

The leader asks the resident to help the others; "Come in and show the others what you are doing. What are you making?" flatters him, since perhaps he feels the sample craft shown him is never made as well as he could make it. Men who have spent their lives in fields and in factories make rugs of simple baling twine of which they're proud, a craft related to an old skill.

Door Mats

EQUIPMENT: Several bushels of scrap baling twine, such as farmers discard.

Procedure:

1. Three varying lengths of scrap baling twine are used to start with.

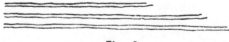

Fig. 8

2. Ends are turned under.

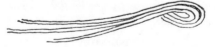

Fig. 9

3. A fourth length of baling twine is wound around the three lengths for about 3″, securing the turned-under ends.

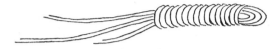

Fig. 10

4. This is curled into a circle and lashed together every sixth time around. The craftsman continues wrapping the winding strand around the three strand core.

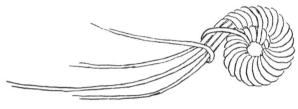

Fig. 11

5. As splicing is needed, another strand is added to each of the core strands, always adding strands of varying length to avoid a weakening in any one place. Splicing is done by separating the ends of the strands, pushing them together, and twisting them into a continuous strand. Care must be taken to make the rug lie flat as one works on it.

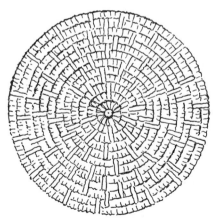

Fig. 12

The Introduction of Something New to an Oldster

First the leader wants to be sure the crafts offered a resident give him a chance to assert his approval and response. The leader tries to understand the reasons he feels useless and help him look at himself. He makes sure the resident will feel accepted and that the activity isn't competitive — crafts which he chooses rather than the leader's choice, are best. He must never appear foolish or embarrassed even to himself, which he may fear will happen if the leader is too domineering.

Perhaps he lets the reluctant resident sit for a while and watch the others enjoying the fun of using their hands. Soon he may say, "I feel good-for-nothing among all these busy people. If they can do it, I can, too." There are many skills which would be difficult to learn in old age, but which people who have learned them earlier in life and who are physically able, enjoy.

Crafts Made from Salvage Materials or Low Cost Crafts

Illustrated crafts at the end of this section show many crafts made of these salvage supplies.

BOXES. To make jewel boxes, crafters spray the inside of a cigar box with felt and cover the outside with tile mosaics or macaroni. Residents do a neat job pasting wall paper on cardboard boxes, covering long adhesive tape tubes to be used for knitting needles, making gift boxes with holiday wrapping paper and fancy boxes for dresser drawers.

MATTRESS TICKING, DISCARDED BEDSPREADS, OR DRAPES. Three B's (Brook's Busy Bees) have a daily coffee klatsch, weave rugs, have officers and a treasury. New mattress ticking donated by a mattress company is used in weaving durable, attractive rugs; part of the money from the rug sales goes to the club, part to the weaver.

DISCARDED NECKTIES.. A woman makes pillows from a variety of men's discarded silk neckties or cuts the ties into small squares making lap robes, sorting out acceptable neckties in good repair for men's bingo prizes.

SWATCHES OF NEW DRAPERY SAMPLES. Samples of new drapery

materials donated by an interior decorator who knows they will be put to good use in the Home, can be made into pillows, stuffed with clipped, discarded stockings or foam rubber. A small nursing home starting a craft program made $60.00 in two months' time by making pillows which the residents sold for $1.00 apiece and which cost them nothing.

Purchase of two washcloths designed with beautiful, large, colored flowers, stuffed with foam rubber and stitched around the edges with rickrack, make washable elbow pillows for the Home or suitable pillows for a child's nursery.

From swatches of large pieces of new drapery material, individual laundry bags are made for each room or are made into smaller disposal bags for wheelchairs and beds. Upholstery or drapery samples make attractive shopping bags; tiny samples of calico on a paper backing are pinked and cut into bridge tallies, sold for a penny apiece or given as gifts.

OLD 78 RPM VICTROLA RECORDS. Old 78 RPM Victrola records heated on a cookie sheet in an oven or in an electric frying pan set at 350 degrees and handled with asbestos gloves, are put in a pail of cold water while they are still hot, the edges ruffled and twisted by hand. Sprayed with white enamel when cool, they look like china plates the edges being painted with gilt and centered with a corsage for a wall plaque. This craft has the disadvantage of needing preparation by the activity aide, however.

DISCARDED DETERGENT BOTTLES. A craft leader suggests calling the nearest laundromat for discarded detergent bottles which might be used in the craft shop; detergent companies will send an illustrated catalogue of an assortment of crafts that residents can make from these containers for the Home — toothbrush holders, bases, toilet brushes, Easter baskets, letter holders, sewing bags and so on.

SHEETS OF CELLULOID OR PLASTIC. Etching is done on a sheet of celluloid, a picture traced on with a pen or a phonograph needle in the end of a 4″ wooden dowel and dots and dashes used for shadings; one can easily shade to correct mistakes. Residents print covers for the Home newsletter, greeting cards, or frame pictures or finished etchings.

Equipment:

1. A phonograph needle in the end of a 4″ wooden dowel to be used as a pen.
2. A sheet of celluloid or plastic.
3. Printers ink, oil or water.
4. An old washing machine hand wringer.
5. Some paper and old rags.

Procedure:

1. The design to be copied is put under the celluloid.
2. The design is scratched into the celluloid with the pen.
3. Ink is rubbed into the scratched design with a cloth.
4. Ink is then wiped off surface, left in scratched surfaces.
5. The paper is wet, then laid on the etched, inked celluloid.
6. It is then run through the washing machine roller on the inked surface, thus making a print of the etching.

IV Tubes. An infirmary uses colored plastic IV tubes broken in half-inch pieces and dyed by cooking with Putnam's dye. The colored pieces decorate detergent containers which take good finger motion to paste on.

Magazine Pictures. A picture in color cut from a magazine pasted on a cardboard is covered with gauze and sprayed with several layers of colorless plastic, resembling an oil painting when it is finished and framed.

Building Tile. Heavy building tile decorated on the smooth surface side makes acceptable bookends which will stand alone.

Burlap, Felt, Weeds and Shells. Residents tack or glue colored burlap to bristol board, glue on a variety of colored flowers made of scraps of plastic and felt, add a bouquet of gilded weeds or starfish and shells which a volunteer brings back from a trip South.

Crafts Purchased in a Kit and Others[1]

Assembly Kits. A Bild-it® kit of precut bird houses, bird feeders, spool racks, spoon racks, pipe holders, doll cradles, bread

---

[1]See pages 346-348 for addresses of craft supply houses.

trays and other items easy to sand, stain, paint or wax and assemble with nails or glue, is a type of assembly kit; completed without carpentry tools, it doesn't require any special strength of hands or arms and makes an item useful and attractive. Assembling and painting plastic birds and animals for planters, model cars, boats or other machines with simple assembling parts, may be of interest as an item for a child's toy or for a whatnot shelf.

LEATHER WORK. Occasionally, men lace mocassins, simple coin purses, comb cases, or purses which are precut, the holes punched complete with snaps, and which are easily laced with a lacing needle.

Scrap leather can also be used for bookmarks. Usually aged and infirm people lack enough strength in their fingers and hands to tool or carve leather, but leather kits which provide a lacing project prove interesting work.

HOBBY GIFT OF THE MONTH CLUB mails a new craft each month for six months, $5.99 post paid — stained glass, crushed stone mosaic, puppet craft, mosaic tiles, colored sand and seed-growing.

MARBLE JEWELRY. Marbles heated in a frying pan to intense heat and then dipped in water crackle into beauty and are put into earring or bracelet settings purchased from a craft catalogue.

CERAMICS. Although not purchased in a kit, ceramics do need special equipment — kiln, heat controls, molds and glazes; a kiln which will fire large ceramics costs from $144.00 on up. Forms may be purchased which make for acceptably turned-out pieces— Santa Claus mugs and poinsettias for Christmas glazed in bright colors are easily marketable, and varieties of dishes, vases, large ash trays, clowns, religious figures, etc., have been popular in craft sales.

Free style ceramics are of even more value therapeutically, of course, as they have creative aspects; and interesting molded heads glazed and successfully fired serve as paper weights, objects of art or whatnot; ash trays seem to be successful with odd shapes suggesting something modernistic and interpretive. Working with kilns requires an activity aide experienced in this craft. There are clays which harden within a few hours or a few days and which will take glazes so that kilns are not always necessary. Some glazes don't require firing.

OTHERS. Aluminum etching, bead looms, braiding, candle making, cane, carving, chenille craft, copper enameling, cork-craft, crystal craze kits, cutting boards, glass etching, handbag kits, hat kits, looper craft, moccasin kits, origami (folding paper into mobiles); number painting, plastic molds (using plaster); raffia kits, reed kits, silk screening (residents don't always like the smell of turpentine); stonecraft (stone chips to make wall plaques); textile painting, wood items to be decorated, wood-burning (to be used with caution); wood stick crafts (popsickle sticks) — besides limitless selections of women's handiwork.

Art Classes

Forming a Sketching Class

The efforts of the residents' art class are tacked at a wheel-chair level in a basement hallway through which residents and employees pass and where sketches can be reviewed. An art show might mean other things — open house or a tea for friends from the community. At any rate, the work is the work of the resident, every stroke his; no indignity to him has been made by touching it up. "We're interested in the patient, not the prod-uct," one tells him.

Each Friday a smiling young woman enters a Home with a pile of "easels" — ordinary wooden breadboards about fifteen by twenty inches on which is tacked clean newsprint for sketching; several boxes of colored chalk crayons are enough for two people to share; and there are items to arrange in a display: fruit, a backdrop, a wooden bowl, a candelabra with six candles and a dozen pieces of wax fruit. Eight women greet her with smiles and pleasant good mornings, exclaiming over her pretty red sweater, she exclaiming over the new dress two of them are cutting out on a table. Two men are escorted in, one eighty-two-years-old and totally deaf, "to watch" the volunteer and the silent women busily working.

The display is arranged; the seated residents take out crayons and tackle the subject.

The young woman says, "Try a circular motion for the round

wooden bowl and the little circles for the grapes, bigger circles for the oranges and apples, straight lines for the candles." In a few minutes forms develop on the newsprint — a yellow banana,

TABLE XIX

BEGINNING NEED WORD LIST[3]

(for Aphasic Patients) (see page 210, "Mounting Pictures," etc.)

A	apple		coffee		hat	O	orange		stocking
	arm		comb		house		....		stove
	ash tray		couch		....		....		sugar
	....		cup		....		....		suit
	....		....		....	P	pajamas		sweater
	....		....	J	juice		pants		....
B	banana		....		....		pen		....
	bathroom	D	dining room		....		pencil		
	bathtub		dish		....		pillow	T	table
	bed		doctor	K	key		pills		tea
	bedpan		dog		kitchen		pipe		teeth
	bedroom		door		Kleenex®		plane		telephone
	belt		dress		knife		plate		television
	Bible		....		....		pocketbook		tie
	blanket		....		....		potatoes		toast
	book		....		....		Prayer Book		toilet
	boy	E	ear	L	lamp		purse		toothbrush
	bottle		egg		leg		....		toothpaste
	box		eye		living room		....		towel
	bread		....		....		....		train
	brush		....		....	R	radio		tray
	bus		....		....		refrigerator		tree
	....	F	face	M	magazine		Rosary		....
	....		feet		matches		....		....
	....		fingers		milk		....		....
C	cake		flowers		Missal		....	U	underwear
	cane		fork		money	S	salt		urinal
	car		....		mouth		sandwich		....
	cards		....		....		shirt		....
	cat		....		....		shoes	W	wallet
	chair	G	girl		....		sink		washcloth
	church		glasses	N	newspaper		slip		watch
	cigar		....		nose		soap		water
	cigarette		....		nurse		sofa		window
	clock		....		....		socks		....
	closet	H	hair		....		soup		....
	coat		hand		....		spoon		....

[3]Compiled by Jan Stovall, Speech and Hearing Consultant, Wisconsin State Board of Health, Division of Chronic Disease and Aging.

green leaves on the grapes. Not a single line is done by the volunteer. The eighty-two-year-old, who can hear nothing of what is said, watches, is urged to pick up the chalk and try some circles of the right color. In a few minutes the man with him begins and they work silently, until the eighty-two-year-old tires and asks to go back to his room. His drawing is put on his closet door with masking tape; he says, "I know what that is for. It is to use time." They tell him, "Yes, and come down next Friday, and we'll do it again."

DRAWING AND PAINTING FREE HAND. A paralyzed young man of twenty-two in a wheelchair who has the use of only two fingers, a thumb, and some shoulder muscles, won third place in a state wide newspaper cartoon contest. With special lessons from a local artist, he now does portraits in oils largely sketching from photographs, and he copies old masters so skillfully he sells everything he paints.

An arthritic walking with two crutches, her hands crippled, is still able to clutch a paint brush to do lovely water color bouquets or Wisconsin red barns which she exhibits in city art shows.

MOUNTING PICTURES AND PRINTING SIGNS FOR USE IN REHABILITATION (working with aphasic patients under direction of the speech therapist). Former engineers, draftsmen, artists or just people who like to draw letters are useful chairmen responsible for the bulletin boards, making signs used in games and quizzes or large recipe signs for the cooking class.

The speech therapist has often asked residents to cut out pictures and label inch-high signs; aphasic patients (unable to talk) can point to these words as a step in making their needs understood and as a step in relearning to speak.

Making Holiday Decorations

Residents make monthly table center decorations or tray favors, trim holiday bulletin boards and windows or make party paper hats. Seasonal patterns from women's magazines, stapler, paints and brushes, colored construction paper, bits of jewelry and buttons, scissors, paste, needle and thread, sequins, gilt braid, yarn, colored spray, cotton, feathers, wooden beads, paper clips, dried and dyed weeds can all be put to use. "Dump all this stuff on a big table and let them go to work," someone has said, offering total creativity for the stiff fingers, creativity which prods residents' ribs and produces a chuckle as they work at these incongruities. Paper hats, party decorations and party supplies can keep a craft shop busy from one holiday to the next.

A valuable volunteer is a teacher who comes in evenings or weekends from the vocational school craft shop, the art class or kindergarten. Perhaps the volunteer den-mother or housewife who likes making her own Christmas presents and redecorating her kitchen every spring can keep a craft shop bubbling with her initiative and resourcefulness. Since some crafts take more than one session to complete, the activity aide makes the sample craft, starts the group on the project, then leaves residents who can continue by themselves while she expands projects in other areas. To avoid spending too much time in craft shops which are open all day, every day, she may assign two dependable volunteers in valuable time-consuming jobs, threading needles, finding supplies, encouraging and making suggestions to busy residents, escorting wheelchairs, etc.

CHRISTMAS CRAFTS. Christmas crafts may be sold at a coordinating council counter which might be Mental Health, Easter Seal or Aid to the Blind, the money from the sale going into the activity fund; crafts made of salvage material or minimum cost items include painting and gilding milkweed pods, seed mosaics on wood, weaving silk stocking rugs on a flat table loom, Christmas angels of gold paper, glittered bells from cardboard egg cartons and painted pine cone trees for table favors.

Residents work on crafts for weeks before the season starts. As well as making Christmas treats in the cooking class, they make nylon net trees, Christmas aprons, plastic Bible covers, school bags, tote bags, Christmas tree skirts, pajama pillows, card table covers of salvage plastic, bibs of finger tip towels, block printed luncheon sets and original Christmas cards of starred Scotch tape on bright colored paper; each resident takes a bell, three and wreath made in the craft shop to his room.

The fancy Christmas bordered aprons are made of one yard of forty-eight inch fabric, for about $1.19 a yard in any department store.

Tote bags woven on a table loom (18″ x 20″ long) are equipped with strong braided handles and fringed tops.

Eleven-inch dolls are completely costumed in knit dresses and caps to match, evening gowns, miniature underwear items and pajama sets.

Gummed tags labeling each craft item reads "A by-product of the activity therapy in .... Home."

Christmas Tree

EQUIPMENT: Construction paper or exposed x-ray film, wire coat hanger, wire cutter and pliers, scissors, glue, ruler, glitter, nail, size of coat hanger wire, hammer and a piece of wood about 4″ x 4″ and ½″ thick.

Procedure:

1. A piece of coat hanger wire 8″ high is cut.
2. A nail hole is made in the center of the piece of wood, so that the coat hanger wire fits tightly into it. The piece of wire is pushed into the nail hole.
3. Strips of paper or x-ray film are cut the sizes indicated, 1½″ wide: ten 10″ strips, nine 8″ strips, five 6″ strips, three 5″ strips, and seven 4″ strips.
4. A hole ¼″ from the end of each strip is punched.
5. The strips are doubled and slipped over the wire, starting with the longest ones at the bottom and graduating them to the smallest ones at the top.
6. The top of the wire is bent in a loop with a pliers, to hold the strips down.
7. Glue is put on strips, lightly sprinkled with a dusting of glitter.

Macaroni Wreath

EQUIPMENT: Macaroni (bow, shell, spiral and ordinary shapes); grout or Elmer's glue; string; heavy cardboard; knife or razor; white enamel spray and a tongue depressor.

Procedure:

1. A cardboard wreath shape is cut with a knife or single edged razor blade. This one is 10½″ across, with a 4″ hole.

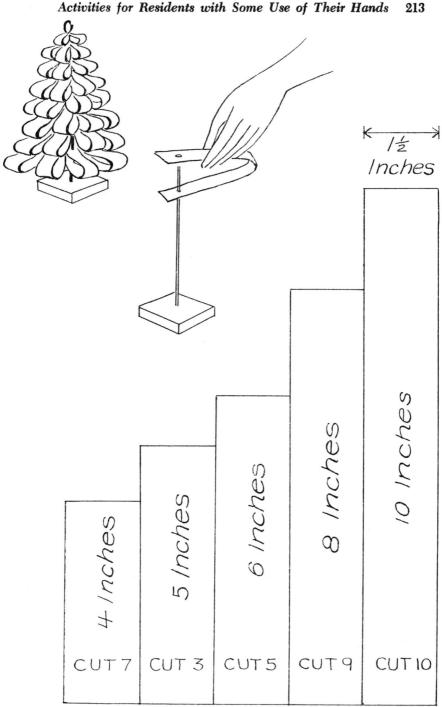

Fig. 13

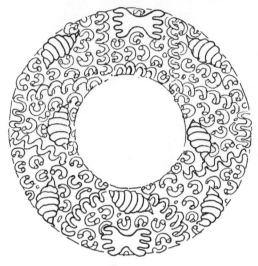

Fig. 14

2. A string loop 1″ from the outer edge is attached.
3. Grout is applied about ⅛″ thick with a tongue depressor to a small area of the cardboard. (Elmer's glue may be used instead.)
4. Macaroni is pressed into the grout without any special design.
5. Front and back of the wreath is sprayed with white enamel when dry. (Residents should not be allowed to use the spray, as it is toxic and should be applied outdoors.)

Jeweled Trinket Box

EQUIPMENT: Miniature plastic cigar box; assortment of fancy

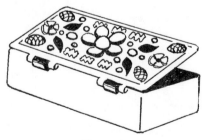

Fig. 15

buttons and costume jewelry; Elmer's glue and gold spray paint.

Procedure:

1. The box is sprayed inside and out and dried.
2. Buttons and jewelry are glued on.

More Decorations

Cardboard shaped like a church window covered with greeting cards, resembling a stained glass window, is used as a wall plaque.

Cattails are painted bright colors to stick in winter bouquets. Using pie tins (foil-ware for freezing), the residents make Christmas wreaths, the fluted edge cut with a tin snip and rolled into loops set close together around the edge of another pie tin.

Cardboard spindle cones (from a stocking factory) and a styrofoam ball for a head make a Christmas caroler, green felt covering the cone for the body and a green felt cape fitted over it. The pipe-stem-cleaner hands hold a sheet of Christmas music.

Residents decorate plastic spoons as Christmas tree ornaments, make snowflake-like designs of cutout plastic strawberry boxes, make table or tray mats trimmed with Christmas cutouts, festoons of paper beads (wallpaper is cut in a 5″ triangle, rolled on a steel knitting needle into a long "bead," and the small end of the triangle is pasted to hold the roll together) to hang on the Christmas tree branches.

Popcorn unsold at a city stand is given the Home where residents color it with vegetable dye and string it for tree decorations. Residents have made a variety of window decorations: fruit jar rubber rings are covered with bits of felt, berries, holly leaves, beads, sequins or stars for miniature wreaths on the tree, trays or the doors; starched net is cut in squares, diamond shapes or ovals covered with sequins and snow men are made of cotton.

Another Home makes ceramic Christmas tree decorations. Clay is rolled out with a rolling pin and cut in designs with a cooky cutter; a hole is punched out with a knitting needle, the ceramic ornament glazed and fired and a ribbon tied in the hole in each to hang on a branch. An inexpensive "experimental" kiln with directions for firing ceramics can be purchased for twenty-four dollars.

In putting up holiday decorations, one must avoid using paste, glue, or Scotch tape on wood paneling, walls or ceramic tiles since it pulls off the paint and will certainly put the committee in charge in bad graces with the matron or superintendent. Masking tape is serviceable and harmless; but decorations ought to be cleared with the person in charge, details discussed regarding fire hazards as well as wall decorations, the use of thumb tacks and moving heavy objects along the floors (or allowing Christmas tap dancers on the newly polished floors).

HALLOWEEN DECORATIONS. Paper hats, noise-makers made of wooden blocks and tambourines made of pie tins and bottle tops all can be made by residents.

Wall decorations for the dining room and recreation room parties might be large black witches cut out in silhouette in different sizes, brooms (cutout or real); witches' hats cutout in cardboard silhouette and painted; paper jack o'lanterns in alternate colors and strung out across the wall or used as mobiles hung from the ceiling; false faces made out of paper maché and painted in gory colors and hung from ceiling or on the wall (two together make for a two-headed effect); black cats' eyes can be painted green and orange with luminous paint on some and pipe cleaners for whiskers; pumpkin heads mounted on broomsticks and hung on walls or around posts; scarecrows, a good way to disguise a post; mobiles: cardboard skeletons, a witch, mask, doughnut, apple, lantern or broom hung where they will have room to turn and twist.

For favors or ceramic pins: clay is cut in the shape of pumpkins, cats, bats, masks, owls, witches' hats or ghosts; or butter cookies made in the cooking class with the dough cut in these shapes can be used for favors.

Safety first! No decorations of paper, leaves or straw unless they are fireproofed! No bonfires without the fire department's permission! No lighted candles or torches!

DECORATIONS FOR EASTER. Residents help make table favors, dye eggs or decorate styrofoam eggs and make Japanese cherry blossom trees by tying bits of pink crepe paper on tiny branches; flowers; ribbons and other suitable material are used for trimming

Easter bonnets which women residents model and for which they receive prizes for the gaudiest, funniest, most elaborate and most feminine.

Crafts for Men

POPSICKLE-STICK CRAFTS. Hawaiian planters are made of ice cream sticks (sometimes 10,000 sticks can be purchased from a local ice cream factory for four dollars) and stained with a variety of wood stains in the craft shop. A small planter can be made with forty sticks (the large size uses seventy pasted together edge to edge with Elmer's glue; or other items can be made such as a small box for cigarettes, jewelry or small trinkets, little fruits baskets, birdhouses and letter holders.

MAKING FURNITURE, CHILDREN'S TOYS AND INLAID BOXES. Any man who has ever used a tool-kit and has the use of his hands, whether or not he's in a wheelchair, can be made productive and happy in some area where noise and dirt are permitted. Basement areas or one end of a maintenance shop in the Home have proven havens for amateur carpenters who make Christmas lawn decorations, children's toys and doll furniture. Even with only two fingers on one hand residents have spent hours sanding precut breadboards or refinishing furniture.

A resident made an easel for a friend working on an oil painting. One of the residents invented a handy holder for the hot cups of coffee from the machine in the Home basement, another, rotating bird feeders to provide a bird with shelter from the wind.

In one Home, the open shelves in the carpentry shop bear the residents' names in wooden letters cut with a coping saw. A former institution laundry has been entirely turned over to carpentry, the medicine ball hanging from the ceiling given an occasional punch in idle time by a passing "carpenter."

It's advisable to post a schedule on the wall of the carpentry shop on which the residents can sign for working hours to prevent a hobbyist from monopolizing the shop and becoming so possessive that he keeps his shoes and socks there and resents anyone else who enters or uses the area.

A complete power workshop in one compact portable unit is basically a fifteen inch jigsaw with a unique power take-off which connects other attachments. It converts to a disc-sanders, grinder, rubbing wheel and flexible shaft which handles as easily as a pencil. It carves, drills, polishes, sharpens, grinds and engraves.

Patterns are available perhaps from the local vocational school or highschool industrial arts class or a state college which teaches industrial arts. A local industrial arts teacher who could spend a Saturday morning or two hours some evening at a regular time can with a few tools, stimulate and direct a few men to a good start in a new hobby area. A simple tool kit with wood files, a saw, a hammer, assorted nails, a vise, shellac and paint would be a start; the appeal of repairing or refinishing furniture in the Home might begin more ambitious carpentry.

Patterns for large furniture items are available. Supervision should be given these areas for certain hours of the day when the areas and equipment are used; if they are electric tools, safety guards should be adapted.

A resident says:

> I have no patterns; all my doll and children's furniture are of my own design and the inlaid woods are my own patterns. To make inlaid boxes I draw a design on a white cardboard, using a ruler and making it perfectly accurate; then I cut and paste the inlaid wood on the cardboard fitting it in perfectly, glueing the pieces together. When it's dry, I soak away the cardboard and have the perfect inlaid piece. I buy seven types of veneer wood from a craftman's wood service company and sell the inlaid boxes to a department store. I've thrown away my crutches!

Some furniture comes ready to assemble.

A resident makes delicate plywood Christmas tree figures cut with a coping saw, and a blind resident has refinished driftwood for centerpieces. Others make step-ups or children's toy boxes, lawn swings, picnic tables and benches and boxes for the outdoor PA amplifiers.

Bird Feeder

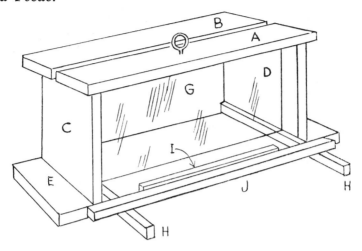

Fig. 16

EQUIPMENT: Seven pieces of scrap plywood or boards:
a roof of two pieces 10″ x 2¾″ (A and B);
back of 7½″ x 3½″ (G);
7½″ x 1⅝″ (F);
bottom 10″ x 3½″ (E), and
two sides 3½″ x 3¾″ (and D).

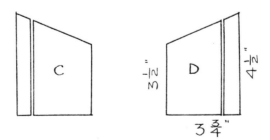

Fig. 17

One ¾″ screw eye, for top; two smaller screw eyes for hook; one 1½″ hook; paint or stain; brush; finishing nails; hammer and saw; glass 8⅛″ x 3¼″.

Procedure:

1. Screw eye is attached to center of **A**, ¼″ from edge.
2. Screw eye and hook are attached to underneath side of **B**. Piece **F** is nailed to underneath side of piece **B**, protruding ¼″.

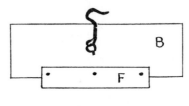

Fig. 18

3. Groove is rabbeted out for glass 1″ from front of side panels on the inside.
4. All the parts are painted or stained.
5. Sides and back to bottom **E** are assembled, the two short side perches nailed to bottom and sides.
6. Front perch **I** is attached to front of bottom piece so that it is ¼″ higher than floor, to keep seeds from falling out.
7. Front perch **J** is added.
8. Glass is put in place.
9. Front of roof is nailed to sides **C** and **D**.

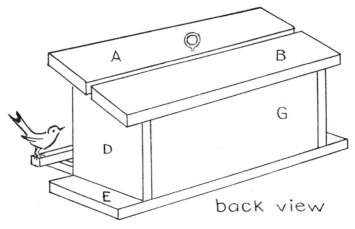

Fig. 19

Note: Roof piece **B** is left unattached so that it may be removed to put in bird seed. Then it may be hooked in place. The feeder is hung near a window and its occupants watched.

Cheese Board

E QUIPMENT:

> A 7" x 7" piece of ½" lumber.
>
> A 7" x 7" piece of formica.
>
> A ½" lumber for other parts.

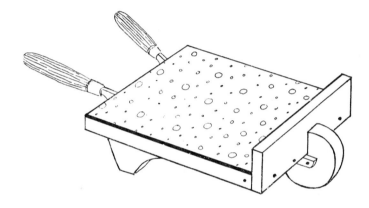

Fig. 20

Two new steak knives (purchased); finishing nails; hammer; saw; sandpaper; Elmer's glue; varnish and brush.

Procedure:

1. The formica is glued onto the 7" x 7" board.
2. The five pieces are sawed out — patterns are on the following page.
3. Grooves for knives in the two backrests are sawed to fit the knife blades.
4. Parts are glued and nailed together.
5. The cheese board is sanded and varnished.
6. The steak knives are placed in the grooves to serve as handles for the little wheelbarrow.

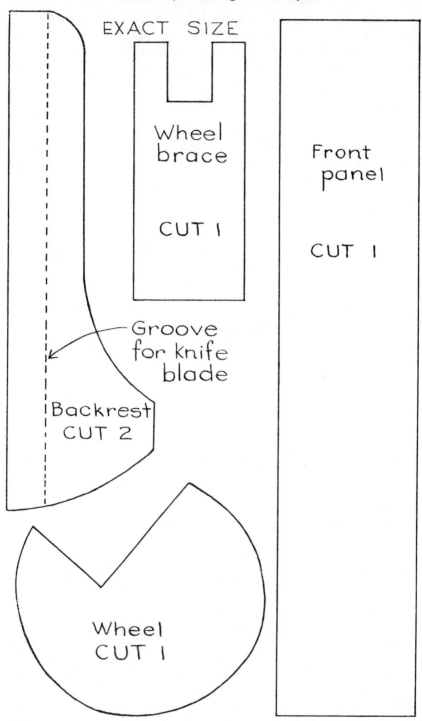

EXACT SIZE

Wheel
brace

CUT 1

Front
panel

CUT 1

Groove
for knife
blade

Backrest
CUT 2

Wheel
CUT 1

Fig. 21

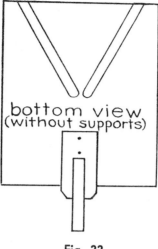

bottom view
(without supports)

Fig. 22

A Home yearly pre-Christmas craft sale, largely of carpentry items, amounted to a sale of $1000.00 worth of crafts. A resident who learned the skill in his youth makes wooden puzzles in dozens of intricately fitted wooden pieces, some in the shape of battle ships.

The plaque posted in a rock garden in another Home has a verse, each letter of which is cut with a coping saw, gilded, and nailed on the plaque.

Ex-President Eisenhower sent a letter of thanks to a resident who sent him a hand-carved plaque. (The resident explained that he had made "Ike's" acquaintance in a chance conversation when the President was on a fishing excursion in Northern Wisconsin several years before. The resident did not recognize the President at first.)

MAKING PICTURE FRAMES. Men make picture frames with the use of a vise, coping saw, hammer and glue, selecting one of a dozen types of wood frame strips to make frames to order.

BUILDING A BOAT AND AN ICE FISHING SHANTY. These unusual accomplishments were achieved by two men in wheelchairs, one with only slight use of his hands, not even enough to accomplish a painting motion; but he designed a twelve-foot boat, counter sunk and fiberglass, with a drop door at the back through which someone could wheel his chair and seat him in the boat. A holder which he drilled at the top of the side held his fishing pole. As the boat was nearing completion, people in the Home wondered whether or not it could be brought up the basement stairs, since there were no windows in the area where it had been built — the resident had planned everything so carefully that there wasn't an extra inch to spare. One wondered if it would float because of its unusual type, but it did; and the two, the helper who had done the sawing and painting and the designer, spent many happy afternoons on the river, once catching a thirty-six inch muskie.

The next autumn found them making a collapsible fishing shanty on runners for ice fishing in the winter. The twelve foot house which has a place for making coffee can be dismantled and stored and was also built in the basement of the Home.

REPAIRING TOYS FOR TOTS. Men residents accept carpentry as an adult, masculine craft and can usually be brought into a carpentry project if invited to repair toys for underprivileged children in the community at Christmas time. This can be developed as a year-round project if volunteers will bring in broken and discarded toys which need refinishing, glueing and slight repairs usually not involving soldering, except as can be done with liquid solder.

A basement area was developed with work tables and good lighting where resident can be noisy and can litter the floor with shavings and sawdust; literally dozens of repaired and repainted wagons, sleds, doll beds and furniture sparkle like new, wrapped in cellophane ready for delivery.

The residents were first contacted by the county police looking for a project for sixty able-bodied aged residents living here. The county also uses the basement area in the Home for storing the toys repaired by other county groups; the Home gains a great deal of good publicity through the project, which brings people from other communities to the Home delivering toys for repair; volunteer groups from the community reach them this way and see the need for other services. Men's church groups and Boy Scouts spend an occasional evening encouraging more residents to take part and work along with them.

A county police officer who had become familiar with the Farm Home in making trips with the ambulance to the Home, started the "Big Brother Project," a name which has nothing to do with the national incorporated group but is the name for this Christmas project.

A large sign outside the canopied doorway leading down to the old basement reads, "Big Brother Project, Farm Home."

The police officer's personal contacts in collecting toys to give underprivilege families were very successful; some toys were already repaired by community groups and stored at the Home as "headquarters," and some were repaired by the residents there.

Not by soliciting from community organizations but by contacting the public personally, the project of collecting broken toys became so big that the community volunteers and residents couldn't keep up with the repairs, so they stored the toys. Now neighbors take the discarded dolls donated for repair, put on new wigs and make new clothes, buying repair supplies themselves. Women volunteers built an addition on their house and invited the public to see the repaired toys. These tours have helped to publicize the program.

The Farm Home remodeled a basement area into a recreation room a year ago when the project was started.

The public has donated between $3000.00 and $4000.00 in tools, plumbing, heating and pipes and has furnished electrical materials and building materials for the walls and floor. The Home had planned to build a room in the basement of this eighty-year-old building, but with this equipment and help, they now have one workshop and six display rooms. Organizations donated a spray booth for painting; tools: a jig saw, a table saw, two joiners, a lathe, hammers and saws; a big awning for the entrance and a sign for outside. Hopeful of getting more and more of these residents working, the Home has a few more come down each week to repair the toys and if nothing more, to clean up or assist in some way.

MAKING VIOLINS, CARVING WOOD AND WHITTLING. Former violin makers with working space and proper lighting can often continue producing instruments as good as ever. A closely related art, wood carving, is possible for people who have strong hands and the wood chisels with which to work. Balsa wood or other soft wood may be preferred, but even wood from the woodpile has been successfully used. Do-it-yourself kits contain miniature totem poles, partially cutout pieces to be debarked, grooved and painted. Blocks of special plaster to be carved can be purchased from craft supply houses. Whittlers have been busy carving miniature wooden shoes, furniture, crucifixes, jumping jacks, miniature farm tools and equipment.

CANING. An infirm man who has never had the use of his crippled legs sits on the floor of a basement shop in the Home and has refinished and caned five thousand chairs in his lengthy stay as resident, an absorbing project, remunerative and physically helpful. A referral to vocational rehabilitation or a local volunteer who canes may give some resident the chance to learn this skill. Instructions come with the caning supplies.

A basement room in one Home has been turned over to a former upholsterer who brought along his tools when he came and who makes time now worthwhile to himself and his customers.

MAKING FISHING FLIES. A volunteer from the city comes in the early spring with supplies: fur, cord, hooks, glue, feathers and ribbon, and instructs men in tying flies. Good vision and strong fingers are necessary in this work, but the flies are easily marketable.

NOVELTIES. Two volunteers from the vocational school work with a group of men who make greeting cards by carving a raw potato as a stamp and make block prints. They also decorate stone paper weights or cover tin cans with mosaics of colored stones the residents have collected.

Many residents are busy shelling hickory nuts, walnuts or butternuts to sell, using a corn husker for some of the hard outer shells.

Crafts for Women

WOMEN'S SEWING PROJECTS. Embroidering, knitting, tatting or crocheting items to sell or give as gifts naturally should have a use; a woman who continues to buy handiwork materials to make more articles only to accumulate them in a dresser drawer finds this discouraging. Sometimes suggestions can be tactfully made as to a change in color or pattern which would make the item more acceptable. Old people often would prefer old familiar skills to something new in the craft shop, such as a do-it-yourself kit or a current handiwork fad.

Sometimes a great deal of importance can be given an item to be used in the Home such as making pillows, wheelchair cushions, dresser scarves and towels. Making their own dresses, mending clothes for others or sewing on name tags is worthwhile and familiar work for the resident.

MAKING HATS. A woman makes calico garden hats and another crochets hats; a retired milliner comes in one afternoon a week for a hat class, redecorating hats with women residents.

DRESSING DOLLS. Occasionally an aged person has made a hobby of collecting antique dolls, making clothing in intricate fashioned detail. Other residents dress fancy boudoir celluloid dolls in dresses of colored circular coffee-filters folded and caught with yarn at the edge. When assembled, the circular filters resemble a full skirt. Four of fifteen women who come to a morning craft shop have had strokes disabling their right sides, and even though all of them were right-handed, they have learned to embroider with their left hand by holding the embroidery firm with metal discs.

To make octopi or pigtail dolls, an 18" piece of cardboard is used on which to wind the skein of cotton yarn, which is then cut at one end to make the strands thirty-six inches long. The center of the skein is then wrapped over a styrofoam ball (the head) and tied tightly together at what will be the neck; the head is decorated with colored felt for the ears and other special features are added and the remainder of the skein is braided and left to hang in eight pigtails which resemble an octopus' tentacles.

Pigtails of braided cotton yarn make pigtail dolls or octopi and also elephants with trunks and large ears made of felt, mice with ears and tails of felt and a bride and groom with veil and high hat or men with four-in-hand ties.

Kleenex Carnation

EQUIPMENT: Kleenex in pastel colors; pinking sheers; fine wire; stiff florist wire; plastic fern and green florist tape.

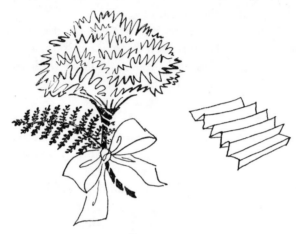

Fig. 23

Procedure:

1. A double sheet of Kleenex is folded in two lengthwise.
2. The whole piece is folded in ½″ accordion pleats and tied with a fine wire around the center.
3. Ends are pinked with pinking sheers.
4. Each layer of Kleenex is carefully pulled apart to make a rounded flower.
5. The ends of the fine wire are attached to a stiffer wire 5″ long for a stem.
6. Green florist tape is wound from the flower down the stem, winding in a small sprig of fern.
7. A narrow ribbon is tied on and a corsage pin added.

Paper Rose

EQUIPMENT: A strip of toilet or tissue paper 36″ x 4½″; fine wire and plastic fern.

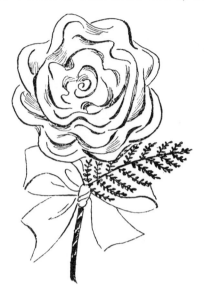

Fig. 24

Procedure:

1. Toilet paper is folded in half, lengthwise.
2. With the fold at the top, the paper is held at the edges and coiled loosely in a rosette shape. The base is pinched together and twisted with fine wire. Fern and stem may be added.

Uses of Paper Flowers: Single flowers may be used for corsages or boutonnieres.

Flowers may be grouped and attached to a large cone of chicken wire for a floral tree. To make an unusual Christmas wreath, wire can be inserted in holes in heavy cardboard and the entire surface covered with flowers. Pale pastels — all pink or all aqua — trimmed with a few small Christmas balls of a contrasting color, make stunning wall decorations.

A large, flat cardboard Christmas tree covered with green Kleenex flowers keeps residents pleasantly occupied for weeks before Christmas and is a most effective decoration for a large wall space for any holiday.

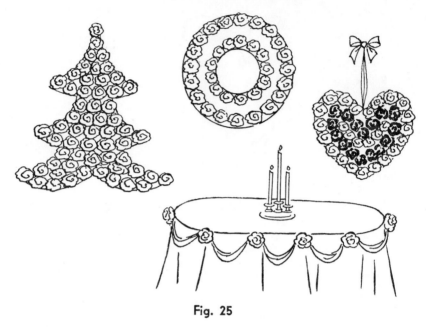

Fig. 25

Flower groupings may also be used for Easter or Valentine decorations, or to decorate the edge of a banquet table in festoons.

Satin Sachet

EQUIPMENT: One yard of wide florist ribbon or satin scraps; one sachet pellet purchased at the drug store; scissors; needle; thread and cotton.

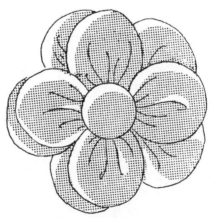

Fig. 26

Procedure:

1. The petal and circle are traced and cardboard patterns are made.

2. Eighteen petals are cut, and two are sewed together around the curve, the straight edge left open. The inside is turned out and straight edge is shirred. Do this with all eighteen petals.

3. Five petals are placed together with edges overlapping and stitched into a circle.

4. Four petals are placed together with edges overlapping and stitched into a circle.

5. The four petal group is placed on top of the five petal group and is secured with a few stitches.

6. Two circles are cut. On one circle a line of shirring ¼" is run from the edge. The sachet pellet is placed in a small wad of cotton (walnut size) in the center of the circle and the stitches are drawn up. This "ball" in the center of the flower is secured.

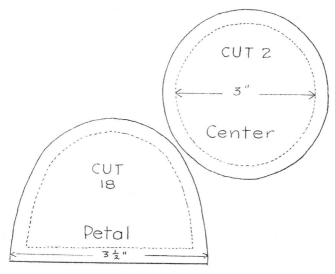

Fig. 27

7. The other circle which has been turned in ¼" and basted is placed on the reverse side of the flower. The bottom of the flower is overcast covering all the raw edges.

Crafts for Men or Women

HUCK TOWELING, EMBROIDERING OR KNITTING. Occasionally men knit their own sweaters or their own socks; an aged amputee in a nursing home knits a sock beautifully in intricate stitches, a sock with a yellow toe and a red heel, for his one foot. A man in his eighties (without spectacles) who does huck toweling and was searching for a bigger project than towels, finally began doing huck embroidery borders on women's skirt materials.

MAKING BRAIDED RUGS. Working at a table in a room is an individual activity, although other residents may assist in preparing strips for braiding, while someone sews the braids. An interesting rectangular braided rug was made with the strips of braid at right angles instead of in an oval.

Sometimes residents sentimentally braid familiar woolen strips from the discarded clothing of friends and relatives.

Nylon stockings braided in thick braids and made to lie flat, wear well and are attractive even in the original gray and biege.

SEWING AND SELLING BALLS OF RAGS FOR RUGS. In many Homes, residents find that morning get-togethers spent tearing and sewing clean rag strips donated by volunteers have been useful and fun. Men and women strengthening their arm and hand muscles with this tearing exercise find that even clumsy fingers can do this simple sewing. Workers happily produced so many balls of rags that they gave the balls to a local weaver, paid her $2.50 for each rug she made with the strips, and sold 140 rugs in one year for three-fifty each, the profit put in an "activity fund" for Home supplies and equipment.

There are many good qualities in this old-fashioned, familiar project for people with "not too good vision and not too good hands"; aged men and women can spend endless evenings and weekends, when no other activity is scheduled, in this pick-up work. It is something to be proud of, a successful and familiar, well-made craft item.

KNITTING ON A CUSTOM LOOM. An infirm resident knits dresses or sweaters, almost any style, color or size, on a loom in his room; some investment is involved; and the cost of new yarn is a consideration, as is learning to operate the loom. But this could become a thriving business; cable-stitch mittens and caps and other very attractive items as well are in great demand. The looms are about $165.00 and will "knit anything that can be knitted by hand."

WEAVING (two harness or four harness looms, rake knitting, etc.). Occasionally residents know how to use a loom or occasionally they will become interested and so are taught the skill; good looms are often purchased secondhand and supplies are furnished by the Home through a revolving fund, the item produced being sold at a small profit to the resident. Other arrangements are made for residents who want to keep the item.

Table mats made on a table loom by weaving two inch strips of plastic dry cleaning bags instead of yarn or calico strips, are less durable but can be used for summer picnics, wiped off, and used again and again.

Physical exercise and satisfaction in achievement are invaluable in weaving; some consideration, however, must be given the fact that only one person at a time can use the loom; and often residents become possessive of it. Colonial loom frames can be made in the carpentry shop and the rake frames used for knitting scarves, stoles, or ropes through an empty spool of thread.

If the activity aide is unfamiliar with the threading of the looms, someone from the craft company from whom the loom is purchased (or the former owner of the loom if it's secondhand) should be asked to help the activity aide in threading it; it often takes two days, and a novice needs instruction. Residents cannot see well enough to do this threading, unfortunately; but an experienced resident-weaver may be able to teach another how to use the loom.

SEWING PINE NEEDLE BASKETS. Able to continue a craft she learned in Florida in her younger days, a resident sews a delicate design in a pine needle basket, proud of a list of orders for more. An Indian resident in another Home makes and can teach this type of pine-needle craft.

MAKING HOOKED YARN PROJECTS (rugs, animals and pillows). Men and women both are interested in hooked yarn if they can make the squeezing motion with their hands which inserts the hook in the burlap, punching the yarn in and out; a frame on which the burlap is spread taut can be laid between two boxes if the resident can stand, but a frame mounted on a standard makes it possible to work from a sitting position. A yarn punch as well as all the other supplies can be purchased at most needle-craft counters in department stores.

Seed Mosaic

Residents with one hand are able to do this craft.

EQUIPMENT: Watermelon, muskmelon, flax, sunflower seeds, corn, tapioca, oats, grain, rice, etc.; plywood; a simple picture from a child's drawing book traced onto the plywood; rubber cement, glue or Elmer's glue and a tongue depressor.

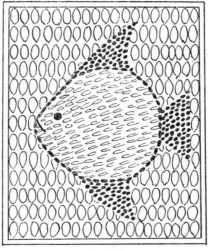

Fig. 28

Procedure:

1. Seeds can be dyed with cold water dyes.
2. With the tongue depressor, a thin layer of cement is spread on an area in which one color is to be used.
3. One type of grain or seeds of one color are sprinkled with fingers or tweezers, covering only the section glued.
4. When this area is dry, another area is glued and seeds of another color used.

Bobby Pin Box

EQUIPMENT: Typewriter ribbon box; scrap felt; 17¼″ gold rickrack; Elmer's glue; variety of sequins and beads.

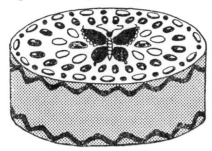

Fig. 29

Procedure:

1. The bottom of the box is traced onto the felt, the two circles cut-out and glued to the top, one to the bottom of the box.
2. A strip of felt is cut 8½″ long and 1⅞″ wide, glued around the side of the box.
3. The rickrack is glued on as well as the sequins and assorted beads for decorations.

Waste Paper Basket

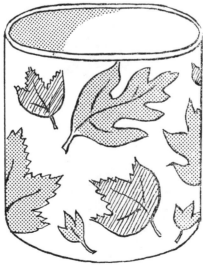

Fig. 30

EQUIPMENT: Leaves; pressed-finish gallon ice cream container; flat white paint; Elmer's glue; 1″ brush; wax paper and an iron.

Procedure:

1. Leaves of different colors or types are pressed in a book or between newspapers and when dried, they are placed between two pieces of wax paper and ironed. Wax paper is removed while warm.

2. The ice cream carton is painted white, both inside and out, and allowed to dry.

3. The leaves are glued to the carton in a pleasing arrangement and allowed to dry.

4. The container is shellaced over the outside for a protective finish.

   This makes a useful, decorative waste basket suitable for any room in the Home.

Tin Can Bank

EQUIPMENT: Pinking scissors; tin can 5½″ x 3¼″; white, blue and green enamel paint; brush; blue and red felt scraps; red or green rickrack 11″ long; a pipe cleaner; scissors; cardboard; artificial leaf or flower spray; ⅜″ bead or pearl for a head.

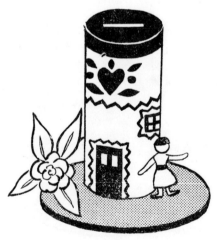

Fig. 31

Procedure:

1. The can is painted with the white enamel.
2. A 5½″ circle of cardboard is cut and painted green for the base.
3. The bottom of the can is glued to the cardboard base.
4. A circle of cardboard 3 and ⅝″ is cut across with a coin slot in it; a circle of red felt is cut the same size and glued to the cardboard.
5. An 11″ x ⅝″ strip of red felt is cut, the slotted circle placed on top of the can and glued on the strip to hold it in place.
6. The rickrack is glued to the can, 3½″ from the bottom.

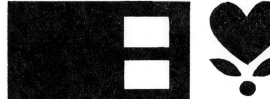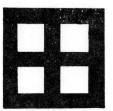

Fig. 32

7. Blue felt door and window frames are cut out with pinking sheers; the door is 2⅛″ x 1½″; window 1½″ x 1½″.
8. Red door and window are glued to the blue frames; blue panes are glued on the red door and window, then these assembled pieces are glued to the can.
9. A small pipe cleaner figure is made with a pearl and bead head, dressed in bits of felt and is glued at the feet and back.
10. A hole in the cardboard is made and the stem of the artificial flower or leaves inserted and glued in place.

Mosaic-Tile Flower Pot

EQUIPMENT: White semi-gloss enamel paint; Elmer's glue; paint brush about 1″ wide; grout (a cement used in laying bathroom tiles); scraps of lightweight linoleum which can be cut with scissors.

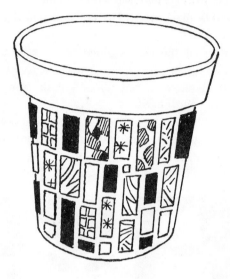

Fig. 33

Procedure:

1. The top rim outside and inside the pot are painted.
2. The linoleum is cut into small squares and rectangles ½″ to 1″ long.
3. Linoleum pieces are glued onto the sides of the pot leaving about ⅛″ between all pieces.
4. When the surface of the pot is covered with pieces of linoleum, it is dried thoroughly.
5. Grout or cement consistency is pressed into all the spaces left between the linoleum pieces. When the grout has dried twenty minutes, excess grout is rubbed or sponged off with a wet cloth, cleaning the linoleum surfaces.

Tile Coaster

EQUIPMENT: Metal top of cottage cheese carton or top of peanut butter jar; pebble-shaped tiles (purchased); grout and glue.

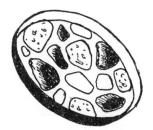

Fig. 34

Procedure:

1. Pebble tiles are glued to inside of lid, ⅛″ apart, and process continued as in the mosaic-tile flower pot, above.

2. If the coaster is to be used as an ash tray, it should be shellacked.

Chapter XIII

ACTIVITIES
FOR AMBULATORY RESIDENTS

Motto: More occupation and less preoccupation.

OUT OF DOORS FOR THE AMBULANT

1. **Games and Activities:** walks, rides, barbecues, horseshoes, croquet and picnics.

2. **Music:** band concerts, barbershop quartets and school choruses.

3. **Hobbies** (outdoor varieties): birdwatching, flower arranging and gardening; card and table games under umbrellas or on the patio; tournaments and exhibits, and club meetings.

4. **Arts and Crafts** (to make outdoors): making costumes for parties; tray favors, handwork, leather lacing, painting toys and play equipment, and other crafts at tables; making outdoor fireplaces and rock gardens, and sketching.

5. **Neighborhood Events:** art shows and exhibits; dog shows, training courses, and holiday observances.

6. **Drama:** festivals, pageants; skits and stunts; judging events; taking part as actors, directors and MC's.

7. **Trips and Package Tours:** to the barber shop, beauty shop, to telephone, to shop, to wayside parks and lake resorts; sightseeing in new community buildings, greenhouses, and florists shops in town; to homes in the community for tea or coffee, to church suppers

8. **Parties and Social Events:** box suppers, family nights, open house, and lawn parties.

Trips into the Community

A<small>NY</small> resident who is able, likes to ride down an old familiar street in an old familiar town or down a country road; he likes to see the Christmas tree lights on the square during the holidays, the Fourth of July parade, a patriotic celebration during the summer, a rural arts show, a community baseball game, and a thousand things of interest in the world outside the Home. In one off-the-grounds trip, it was touching to hear those residents exclaim who had never seen a Diesel train, never seen a ranch style house, the new court house and all the other changes one takes for granted in everyday life.

If the Home has a Home-owned station wagen or bus, fine; but before the activity aide ever solicits volunteers to give rides to residents, he must clear this with the superintendent, who may have to clear it with the trustees, or other people to whom he's responsible. In some Homes, the volunteers must sign the residents out, which means they take full responsibility for them; sometimes a permit signed by the nearest of kin of each resident is on file. In most of the Homes, the charge nurse, matron or superintendent verifies the list of residents who want the ride and no trouble has ever resulted (see p. 100).

The subject of volunteers providing cars and taking residents for a drive has come up frequently. One volunteer had her insurance company write in a clause at no extra charge, stating that the owner and driver of the car (and the policy holder) has permission to carry passengers or "guests." The Wisconsin State Insurance Department, Rates Division says that any ordinary insurance will cover this service by volunteers so that no special clause is necessary. "As long as the driver doesn't charge for giving a ride, she isn't liable."

Attending an annual Fall Festival parade, residents are given a ride in an old open Model T Ford driven by one of the clowns.

Shut-in-Day may mean a trip downtown to Library Park at the invitation of a local business group. A hot dinner for the residents served by the businessmen and their wives precedes a program of professional entertainment. A local radio station makes tapes of the annual affair, interviewing residents, and later playing the tape back to the group and again over the radio station. Corsages and boutonnieres are given the guests.

"Seeing things and going places, they have a better idea of what the world is like today with its constant changes. Visiting other aged and infirm people they often feel they're pretty lucky," a nurse says.

WHERE TO GO. The county home bus has taken residents many miles for a day's excursion to see the Dells, a professional game and to the Circus Museum, etc. Shorter trips for an afternoon are easily planned: one Home is given tickets by a local theatre any time residents plan a theater party; others take trips through the paper mills, through their doctor's new medical clinic, the new junior high school, the new fire house or to the voting polls. The local park gives free rides on the miniature train each time Red Cross volunteers take residents on a tour to the park.

Another Home arranges a bus trip for residents, two hours for $10.00, a bus load including forty residents who go sightseeing, visit the airport, a local college or enjoy a lakeside view. A captain from the harbor commission serves as host when they tour a ship in dock; again, they visit a truck farm, see the new high school, an octagonal church of interest, and the shopping center which proves even more exciting. Once after telephoning the florist announcing a visit, each resident was given a corsage at the shop. During the summer, the Home rents a bus from the city bus company which normally transports orthopedic children to school. The Home uses the school bus summer months or weekends when it is not otherwise being used and finds it especially adaptable since the bus has a lift for hoisting wheelchair residents up and into the bus.

One Home has a station wagon which the activity aide herself drives each Friday afternoon, impartially taking residents in turn. Church members sometimes assume the responsibility of picking up fellow church members in the Home, taking them to women's circles, or men's monthly church suppers.

Often residents regularly attend the local Golden Age Club meetings making friends in the community.

Seventeen cars furnished by volunteers in a small town

annually bring residents to a beautiful country home used as a girls' summer camp, where residents spend an afternoon being entertained by the teenagers. The girls, who have spent days making cookies and picking wild flowers for bouquets, entertain the residents in the grape-arbor patio, singing folk songs and playing the cello and the guitar. It's a treat for the aged to see young faces and these sophisticated teenagers from the big city feel a self-importance in assuming the responsibility for the afternoon for some of them have never known grandparents, or indeed, any aged person.

The resident takes pleasure in dressing especially for these trips and he will talk about them for weeks, remembering the smiles, the handshakes and the shared jokes. The beautiful view along the way is often familiar yet ever-changing to oldsters.

Games in the Bus[1]

MILEAGE. At the command "Guess," all players estimate the distance to a point designated: a house, hill, turn in the road or a tree far down the road. The resident who comes nearest to the correct distance as registered by the speedometer, wins.

ROADSIDE POKER. A player watches the countryside for certain objects and scores the following: a white horse, two points; white sheep, one point; white dog, three points; white rabbit, twenty-five points. He shouts, "White dog" (or whatever), but if it turns out to be white sheep, he loses ten points. Other objects, animals, or persons may be substituted.

COUNT-DOWN. Players on one side of the bus, or in the front or back seats of a car, count the number of churches that are passed along the road, in towns as well as in the country. The other side will count the number of school houses or filling stations or drive-ins, playing the game to the destination of the trip.

WHAT LIES AHEAD? Guessing such things as the number of turns in the road before coming to the next town, the number of left turns, and the number of right turns, makes the trip more interesting. Even though it's not visible, the number of windows

---

[1] Taken from **Games for Quiet Hours and Small Spaces.** New York, National Park and Recreation Association. Used by permission.

in the next farmhouse on the right side of the road or anything else about the farmhouse, such as the location of the entrance, the kind of chimney, the color of the house, its flower garden, or lack of one can be guessed. Each person makes his guess and when the house appears, a point is scored for each correct guess. As he plays, each passenger will think up new things to guess about.

GUESSING CARS. Residents in the bus guess the color of the next car, the make of the car, whether or not it will have white-walled tires, etc. Each passenger names a certain make of car, no two players being allowed to select the same kind. Only cars moving in the opposite direction are considered.

OBJECT LESSON. Everyone identifies birds, trees or flowers observed en route during a given trip or in a certain length of time. The player with the greatest number of kinds of objects, wins.

TOURING MEMORY CONTEST. One person starts the game, saying, "I see . . ." mentioning some interesting object observed on the trip. The next player repeats what the previous player saw and adds his own observation; the next repeats the list in the right order and adds something. This can get pretty hilarious.

Picnics

PICNICS. Of the marshmallow roast, they write, The charcoal grills were ready and the service tables arranged, the nursing staff busy seeing that everyone was comfortably seated, when Girl Scouts came in laden with the ingredients necessary for the "Some Mores"; they served a tasty Girl Scout recipe of a graham cracker sandwich filled with a layer of a chocolate bar and a toasted marshmallow.

The girls were kept busy toasting marshmallows and supplying the residents unable to be outdoors. One of the residents was on the run helping others, and not a crumb would he take until everyone had been served. Another man furnished all the sticks, which he whittled from branches he gathered.

Problems of loneliness and residents' reluctance to attend outside affairs are dispelled by each resident inviting a friend, someone with whom to sit at the picnic. In most Homes, families bring their own lunches and the lunch for the resident, the Home furnishing the drink. At the family picnics arranged in the Home which limit free ice cream and pop for children, they issue each child a ticket, so that he gets one treat.

Before the Picnic, the Plan

A committee must be formed for major planning, publicity, and some of this responsibility can be assumed by residents. Written minutes will help in checking on decisions and responsibilities.

THEME. In some years, the theme will be obvious: for example, tenth, fiftieth, or other Home anniversaries; other themes could be Western, Indian, May Day, Memorial Day or Pirate, the theme being carried out in the publicity, in the program, the costumes (like funny old-fashioned hats for everyone), the tickets, the decorations, the games and the prizes.

Where to Hold the Picnic

1. Is there enough room in the area for everyone who will attend?
2. Are there rest rooms within easy walking distance, and electricity if one depends on using it?
3. Are there enough tables and chairs?
4. Is there enough parking space nearby?
5. Is there a sheltered area in case of rain?
6. Is permission to use the area necessary?
7. Is it near enough to the Home?

Doing the Job — Committees at Work

1. Have meal tickets or numbers for drawing, for instance, been previously prepared?
2. Have arrangements been made for attendants or volunteers who are assisting wheelchair residents?
3. Has the kitchen been notified of the definite number who will need lunches?
4. If it's barbecue, what about fuel?

5. Is there someone to take pictures?
6. Are prizes ready?
7. Has a public address system been tested?
8. Have buttons, tags, hats or other forms of identification all been prepared?
9. Is emergency first-aid ready?

PRIZES. A good prize is the best tonic any picnic can have. Prize-winners like to show their prizes to friends, even if they are small and inexpensive.

An appealing way of giving consolation prizes is the treasure chest or wishing-well filled with novelties which each resident may dip in and take as prizes: men's straw and cloth caps, white gob hats, compass, sheriff badge, pirate flag, whistle, key chain, squawker balloons, flying birds that sing, pinwheels, paper lasso that whistles, blowouts for fun and noise, flying saucer, cup and ball, "finger trap" tricks, parasols, rings that glow in the dark, parachute with a doll attached, etc.

Program

BALLOON SWAT. Ten or twelve people standing in a circle to start are given fly swatters or rolled newspapers, and balloons are tied to a piece of string perhaps 3′ or 4′ long. The string is tied around their waists so that the balloons are in back. When the signal is given, they begin swatting each other's balloons, at the same time trying to protect their own. As soon as a player's balloon is broken, he is eliminated from the game.

BALLOON SCRAMBLE. Contestants tie or hold one hand behind their backs and balloons are released. At the end of a time limit, prizes go to residents who have been able to gather the greatest number of balloons with their free hands.

BALLOON BAT. Contestants line up behind a designated spot. At the signal all the players at the same time bat their balloons with open palms across the open space, around the goal and back to the starting line.

BALLOON HIT. Contestants are given balloons and baseball bats or ping-pong rackets. Starting at the same line, they try to swat the balloons across the designated finish line.

BALLOON EMBRACING. Couples face one another, place a ballon between their chests and embrace one another. The couple who bursts the balloon first is the winner.

CRAB KICK. Contestants kick a bag — which won't break and contents of which won't hurt their feet — along the ground in front of them to the finish line. If the bag lands in front of another player, the second player simply ignores the bag and persistently pursues only his own.

SLIPPER KICK. Contestants stand in an even line and loosen the shoes on their kicking feet, freeing the feet so the shoes can be kicked off; those who kick the shoe the greatest distance win.

CRAZY WALTZING. Couples try to waltz back to back with their arm interlocked.

DANCING FOREHEAD TO FOREHEAD. Perhaps a very tall person and a short person face each other, and with a ping-pong ball between their foreheads, they dance a waltz with hands behind them.

MIXING SHOES. Women are seated, shoes removed, mixed and placed in shoe boxes. Boxes are closed and placed in front of contestants. At "go" women find their own shoes and put them on.

PASSING THE EGG. Couples line up with hands behind their backs; a pie tin with a hardboiled egg in it goes under the chin of first contestant, who passes it along to the next one and so it goes from chin to chin without the help of their hands.

TYING APRON STRINGS. Two men wearing aprons stand back to back. The contest is to have each man tie the apron string in a bow tie at the back of the other resident without looking.

WALK AGAINST TIME. Contestants are told they have a certain length of time in which to walk a certain distance. At the end of the specified time, the whistle blows, and the contestants stop where they are. The winner is the player nearest the finish line without yet crossing it.

Gardening

Residents enjoy taking care of winter gardens (sweet potatoes or other vegetables growing in water) or being responsible for summer vegetable or flower gardens. Residents, in the fall, bring in seeds from the flower gardens, package them in varieties of mixed old fashioned flowers, and sell them or give them with a little verse to a friend. One may make rose petal sachets from dried roses in cut flower bouquets brought to the Home or from summer gardens. Pine cones are collected and sprayed for Christmas tree ornaments; greens and cat tails are sprayed, berries and dried weeds and wild flowers are arranged in bouquets. Charcoal filler (hardwood ashes) put in a glass bowl dampened and covered tight with Saran® Wrap, will keep moss and tiny ferns from needing further watering.

Wreaths made from weeds and berries painted with liquid wax will help decorate the Home or can be given as gifts.

Many Homes have greenhouses in which green-thumb residents may assist an employee; an ambulatory resident built his own hot house out of scrap lumber and windows. In a new Home, a waist-high planter forty feet long runs the length of the craft shop, large-paned greenhouse windows slanting out to southern exposure. When a banana tree, six feet high, sported a purple acorn-shaped bud, the practical joker in the Home taped on a ripe banana!

Residents supplied flowers they had raised from seeds for all the table decorations at a city convention. Walking with canes, residents were busy all summer with tomato, cabbage and pepper gardens, even the last few weeks before frost, busily tying up the vines. They brought in five large cabbage heads for cabbage salad one day for the first floor dining room where the gardeners ate. In the evening, when one of the residents heard on the radio that it would freeze, he hobbled out and harvested all the green tomatoes.

One of the service men who makes trips to the Home said, "This is the bright spot of my route, coming up here to see the beautiful flowers the residents have grown."

"Gardening is something they've loved doing," the superintendent says. "I've learned to let a patient do what he wants to do; you can't **make** him do it or you spoil the project for him. We have a lot of projects going on at the same time from which he may choose; recreation means nothing if he has to be made to do it. Next year we'll plow up a big garden, and each resident can have as much room as he wants.

"In the spring one resident had said, 'My hip is too stiff, and my fingers are too crippled to go out there and work,' but when she saw the others, she was out there, too."

When a local Garden Club came, forty residents started bulbs indoors in pots and then planted them outside. The club provides food for bird feeders placed on the shelves outside the residents' windows; this project is being encouraged in garden clubs, promoting the pleasure of bird watching.

Taking Care of Animals and Birds

Deer and other animals are available from the State Conservation Department if the Home has a fenced area, and other requirements are met regarding the animals' care.

Of interest to residents are 3,010 day-old pheasants which come from the state game farm and the Rod and Gun Club. Residents are interested in feeding the pheasants crumbles for the first six weeks and then they give them pellets and lettuce. At the end of the twelve days, the birds are put out in the holding pens, at the end of the twenty-eighth day, in the runways, and after ten weeks, they are moved to another locality better suited to wild life.

Blackbirds are trained to be fed in the mornings in the front yard of one Home and goldfiish come to the surface to be fed by oldsters; squirrels are taught to pick the acorns balanced on the foot of a resident sitting in the yard. A circle of wheelchair residents taught a chipmunk, Mike, their pet for three summers, to come to their laps or perch on their shoulders to pick up peanuts.

Residents enjoy feeding the chickens or doing other chores at the Farm Home.

Miniature Golf

If a large lawn is available, coffee cans set in the ground can be used for the golf cup, and donated balls and golf clubs can make possible a type of miniature golf; pins, tees and a flag designating each hole along with other props can make it a convincing game requiring some skill.

Fishing in an Accessible Area

One of the nursing homes has fishing gear available in the activity aide's office, a pond stocked with fish, a table at the edge of the pond on which to clean the fish and a barbecue to cook them. To assure safety, residents in another Home built the dock where they fished at the edge of the river flowing through the Home property. Several other Homes have nearby streams where residents may walk or be taken by car to spend the day; fishing gear may be donated or cheap bamboo poles for residents' use signed out from the Home activity office.

A load of fish arrives from the State Conservation Department in the spring to stock the pond on the Home grounds for the residents who fish and for the hundreds of youngsters who come out from town to fish with them in the summer.

INDOORS FOR THE AMBULANT

PUNCHING BAGS (medicine ball). Aged men will enjoy a punching bag hanging within reach, perhaps in the craft shop or carpentry area.

GIVING PLAYS. Plays with plots of old-time themes, fun and entertainment which oldsters will enjoy, may be ordered through catalogues or found in Traveling Library books. Residents read the lines from script typed in capitals. In one Home, they gave a play to entertain the employees on Mother's Day, the residents' play rehearsals having been scheduled in the daily programs posted on the bulletin board weeks beforehand.

RESIDENT TALENT SHOWS. There are always a few residents, no matter how aged and infirm, who will recite, demonstrate a card trick, tie trick knots, play a guitar, a fiddle, or a concertina, sing a song they've composed or recite a poem they've written, sing a hymn-duet or tell a joke. Residents often love to perform, especially to a group of visitors, so it's easy to supplement a community group from a dance studio or a barbershop quartet with some resident talent, no matter how often the residents may have seen the performance. Surprisingly, they will come out on crutches, in wheelchairs or leaning against a cane to face a large audience and enjoy it.

Costumes give importance to an amateur production. One Home has collected clown suits, a tux, a formal, a tramp suit, a master-of-ceremonies costume, a bridal gown and other attire in which to dress up and which helps add color to a show. Simple skits typed in capital letters and easily read are rehearsed many times. In one instance a pulpit with a light was used at which each player stood to read his lines.

A resident-chorus practicing with another outside chorus presented a combined concert; joining a stronger group gave them volume and moral support.

The idea for talent shows sprouted in one Home when a rhythm band wanted to put on an hour long program for fellow residents; and as that would have been too much strain for the band alone, they had to find some "fill-in" acts for residents to do.

When the aide discussed this with the band members, one said he had seen a professional singing act and would like to duplicate it if he could have one of the nurses with him; trying to use the talents of the residents, they induced a resident-poet to read one of her favorite poems. There were harmonica players, soloists (one partially mentally retarded resident did very well in this), and to add a bit of humor, one resident who consented to be made-up, dressed as a hobo and used large cue cards instead of memorizing his lines. Several practices made him familiar with proper voice inflections.

Satisfaction the residents derive from performing comes with team spirit, self-confidence and from the applause and acclaim from fellow residents.

A SHORT SHORT contribution to the "drammer club" is this hillbilly skit:

> *As the scene opens, six members of the family are seen silhouetted against the blue-lighted backdrop. They are seated about the stage. Lem, the smallest, has his feet up against the lamppost. There is quiet on the stage, except for the sound of a bottle and an occasional snore. Then there is a terrible baying and Paw comes to.*

PAW. Maw! Hey, Maw! Maw!

MAW. (from right behind him). Here, Paw!

PAW. Go see what that hound dawg's howlin' about, willya? I'd go myself but I'm too tired to move. (**Dog howls.**)

MAW. 'Zekiel! Go see what that hound dawg's howlin' about, willya? I'd go myself, but I'm too tired to move. (**Dog howls.**)

ZEKE. Ezra! Hey Ezra! Go see what that hound dawg's howlin' about willya? I'd go myself, but I'm too tired to move. (**Dog howls.**)

EZRA. Lem! Lemule! Go git yo'seff up and see what that hound dawg's howlin' about willya? I'd go myself, but I'm too tired to move. G'wan now, git! (**Dog howls. Lem rises slowly and stumbles off the stage. Dog yelps in anguish, then Lem comes tiredly back on the stage.**)

LEM. The howlin' dawg is howlin' 'cause he's sittin' on a cactus, and he's too tired to move.

Dancing

A Home newsletter lists the residents who wore formals at the dance:

> The Home had its formal party from 7 PM to 9 PM in their recreation room; many county home residents were there. .... and his orchestra furnished the music. The women wore beautiful formals and the men had lapel boutonnieres. As each couple entered the room they paused at the foot of the stair while the master-of-ceremonies introduced them before they took their places in line — the women on one side, and the men on the other. The King and Queen were seated at the head of the room. When all were in line they took part in the grand march.

Another newsletter reports the following:

> Residents were escorted to a party out of town given by the YWCA for residents by bus and volunteers in private cars. Women received corsages and the men, a small white mum and fern twigs for their lapels. The afternoon was spent in dancing, music furnished by a piano player and one of our own accordion players.

Playing records on a record player will do for dancing, of course, but "live" music is always more fun. If a musician-employee or a volunteer can come in at a regular time to play a musical instrument, a happy social hour follows. Residents unable to dance can keep time with triangles or gourds, serve as judges, march together in a grand march, take charge of the record player, whistle or tap their feet and sing.

Square dancers from the community may be invited to come in to give demonstrations, drawing a few residents into the simpler, less strenuous dances; men-volunteers dance with the women-residents and women-volunteers dance with men-residents. Community square dancers contributed square dance costumes to a Home, and the dresses were kept in a costume room and used only for these affairs. With big groups in a big room, a microphone and amplified music are necessary.

Simple folk dances are possible for any resident who can walk. The following are revised for oldsters:

Folk Dance Calls

Strut, Miss Lizzie[1]

The music is "Shortnin' Bread."

Formation: Two lines facing each other, partners across from each other hold hands.

> 1   2   1   2   1   2
>
> This a-way, Valerie, That a-way, Valerie, This a-way, Valerie,
>
> 3
>
> All the way home.

4   (Repeat)

5   Strut, Miss Lizzie, strut, Miss Lizzie;
Strut, Miss Lizzie, all the way home.

6   Here comes another one, just like the other one;
Here comes another one, all the way home.

Action: 1. Extend one foot forward with heel touching floor.

2. Return foot to place (Alternate feet.)

3. Clap three times.

---

[1] **Eleanore Kaiser,** City Recreation Dept. Sheboygan, Wisconsin.

4. Lines separate, so that there is a four foot space between.

5. Person at the head of the line leaves his place and struts to a new place at the foot of his line. Others clap.

6. First person at the head of the other line leaves place and struts to a new place at the foot of his line. Others clap.

Song is repeated until each player has had a chance to strut. Demonstrate different struts and encourage participants to strut in different ways (like a sailor, like a hula dancer, like a show-off, etc.)

Note: Original instructions called for a hop step on **"This,"** **"That,"** and **"This,"** and a quick succession of three hop steps on "All the way home."

Invented and played in a Home with volunteers, this stunt for exercising the hip and body is shown below.

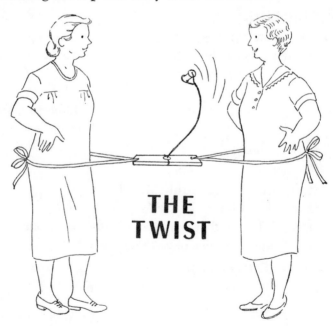

THE
TWIST

Fig. 35

EQUIPMENT: A piece of plywood 12″ long and 1½″ wide; four yards of tape or strips of ticking 18″ long.

Procedure in Making:

1. A ¼″ hole is bored ½″ from each end of the board.

2. The tape is cut in two equal lengths, two yards long and each piece threaded through the hole in the piece of wood.

3. The string is put through the spool and tied in a firm knot. The other end of the string is tied to the middle of the piece of wood.

Procedure in Playing:

1. Strings are tied around the waists of two ambulatory people who face each other with hands on hips.

2. They swing hips to make the string with the spool whirl around the board; several couples can race, which is good for laughs.

Parties for the Recreation Hall

If one of the party activities doesn't seem to be going well, the leader discards it for another time, always sure to have some other activity to fall back on should his plans go over like a lead balloon. Often the success of a party is hard to predict.

The mixer, setting the mood, and party get-acquainted stunts help start the party and can be used anywhere as substitute activity during the party. These stunts may help start residents in activity as they arrive at the recreation hall.

The Mixer — Setting the Mood

THE LEFT-HANDED MIXER. Guests are notified upon entering that all hand shaking must be done with the left hand. A large autograph card and a prize is given for greatest number of autographs secured in twenty minutes. All autographs must be written with the left hand.

WHAT YOU'RE DOING. Three volunteers help; one moves among residents who draw slips of paper on which is written **with whom he is** supposed to be. Two gives him a slip telling him **where he is**, and three **what he is doing**. The leaders, of course, work independently. The group is then assembled and each person states his name, tells **whom he is with, where he** is and **what he is doing.** "My name is Bill Smith. I'm with Baby Snooks at the beach, skiing." If the slips are numbered — all the ones, all the twos and all the threes — the residents will read them in the right order.

GUESS AGAIN. As the resident arrives he is presented with five or six small pieces of paper in various colors and is told to start shaking hands and exchanging slips with other guests. However, he is not told what exchange to make. He is told that in ten minutes the time will be called and slips tallied. Perhaps the resident with all red, or half blue and half green, will win, he is told, but it's up to him to decide; no one knows. The resident is left with a curious feeling — to exchange or not to exchange. When time is called, the results are tallied.

10 points, each red	A black slip cancels the
8 points, each blue	whole score, and one set
6 points, each green	of each color, adds 10.
4 points, each yellow	One set of the same color
2 points, each white	adds 30.

MATCHING PROVERBS. Each man and woman is given half a proverb which he must match at a signal. For variation each woman is given a card upon which a proverb is written and each man is given a card upon which the idea expressed in a proverb is couched in high sounding English. All players circulate and find partners by matching proverbs.

Example: A stitch in time saves nine.

A small one-eyed steel instrument, used at the crucial moment, may rescue the square of three.

Other items may be matched by giving half of the items to women and the other half to men.

Or match up for groups; jig-saw pictures, songs and poems may be used.

TEN BEANS. Each person is given ten beans or other counters and then engages in conversation with other players, being careful not to use the forbidden words, "yes" or "no," or "I," "my," "mine," and "me." Should either resident detect the other using a forbidden word, he will receive on demand, one bean for each offense. Person having most beans wins.

For variation the player challenges other players to guess if odd or even number of beans is being held by him. If he guesses wrong, he must forfeit a bean.

INFORMAL DIALOGUE. As the guests arrive, each woman is given an even-numbered card and each man an odd, the first line of which might read, "You are number six. Please carry out the instructions below." This might be followed by two or more of the items similar to these:

"Find number seven and introduce him to number eleven."

"Find number four and ask her to help you make a list of people with the most hair."

"Find number three and ask him to help you find out how many people have a middle name beginning with a vowel."

SIGNATURE HUNT. Each man who is given a slip of paper containing ten instructions, gets the signature of a woman wearing nail polish — earrings, a comb in her hair, a brooch or something else designated to be found. Each woman given a slip asks for the signature of a man wearing suspenders, a hearing aid, a tie clip, etc.

There must be a different signature on each line. A prize is given to one who can identify all names on his slip. This may also be used later as a mixer by having supper with number five on the slip, etc.

Introduce, after a long build up, Mr. Benjamine McGillucudy who is passed from hand to hand down the receiving line. Benjamine is a rubber lizard.

BIG BUSINESS. Each player has ten grains of corn, beans or peanuts and five paper clips, which, at a signal, he begins trading. He is told that the one with a lucky number of paper clips or beans will win. The player with the most paper clips and beans will also win. Since no one knows the lucky number (which the leader has written on a slip of paper previous to starting), the trading will be regulated by the player's guesses.

Get Acquainted Party Games

A TO Z BINGO. Each resident has a paper with twenty squares, a different letter of the alphabet in each square. Object is to find someone whose name begins with that letter and list it.

NAME BINGO. Each resident has paper with twenty squares. Object is to get a different signature in each square. Each person should deposit his own name in a box provided for that purpose. Names are drawn from the box, as numbers are drawn in bingo game, and players cross off names on the sheets. First one to get five in line wins.

As person's name is drawn from the box, he may raise his hand so all can see and identify the name and face.

SKELETON NAME. Each person has a pencil, a tag with a string and a card. Each player puts his name in skeleton form on the tag, i.e., he writes his name omitting the vowels but marking a dash in place of each vowel. (**Example:** John Newton would be J—hn Newt—n. He fastens the card on himself. Players gather as many names as possible filling in the skeleton.)

WHAT'S YOUR NAME? Everyone has a card and pencil, and vertically down the left hand side he writes his name, first and last, one letter under the other. Residents look through the crowd and find players whose names contain letters corresponding to each one of the letters in his own name: **J** — Judith; **O** — Oliver; **H** — Harry, and **N** — Nancy.

PAPER BAGS. Paper bags are put on each person's right hand. Everyone proceeds to get as many signatures on his bag as he can before time is called.

FAMOUS PEOPLE. The name of a well-known person in history, movies, radio, etc., is pinned on the back of each resident who endeavors to find out who he is by asking questions that may be answered "yes" or "no."

ON THE SPOT. Each person has three counters. At a starting signal, players start a conversation with the person sitting next to him. After a moment the stop signal is given, and everyone stops talking. One red card and one black card which have been prepared beforehand are drawn from the box. The red cards contain the location of the unlucky spot, the black, the lucky. The couple standing nearest the unlucky spot described on the red card must each give a counter to the couple standing nearest the lucky spot.

MAN IN THE MOON. As many round "moons" are cut out as

there are residents, one color for the women, one for the men. Placing two "moons" together, five or six holes are punched with a paper punch, varying the position and number of holes so that no two sets are alike. Players find partners by matching the holes in the moon.

DIME IN THE CROWD. It is announced that two or three people in the crowd are "millionaires" and will pay a huge sum to every tenth person who shakes his hand. Residents shake hands in hopes of finding "millionaire" who will reward them with a dime if they are the tenth person.

Party Stunts

TIME GUESSING. Perhaps a special stunt for the New Year's party would be the clock tied up in paper so that no one knows at what time the hands are set. The resident guessing closest to the correct position of the hands when the package is opened wins the clock or some other prize.

GUESSING GAMES. The number of people in the room, the weight of the committee chairman, the number of pennies in a piggy bank, the number of peanuts in a bag, the length of a ribbon on the box, the weight of a bowl of fruit — everyone can try these games.

BALL TOSSING. Two people toss a ball to one another, each time stepping back a step, perhaps as far as eight or ten steps, continuing to throw the ball until they miss.

ALPHABET LETTERS. Someone calls a simple word to a group of twenty-six people each of whom holds a letter of the alphabet; each person holding a letter in the word called, steps forward to form the word, perhaps in a race with time.

HA-HA GAME. The activity aide or a resident in the group tries to make each person (perhaps lined up on the stage) laugh (like "Poor Pussy," where the player gets down on his knees and pretends to stroke the "cat," rub her ears or something foolish to amuse her).

WHO AM I? A picture of a movie star, TV personality, a famous athlete, or a politician is pinned on someone's back without his knowing its identity. He asks questions of the others in the group trying to identify it, since all others in the group are allowed to see it. This also, works well on a stage where an audience can watch and help with the answers.

Miscellaneous Party Ideas

PRINTED INVITATIONS. A volunteer with a printing press donates special program flyers distributed at affairs in the Home; she also sends residents individual printed invitations for birthday parties: "Shady Lawn volunteers announce a birthday supper in the dining room of Shady Lawn Home (date). . . . . Hope to see you," and lists residents celebrating birthdays.

SPECIAL DIETS AT THE PARTY. People on special diets who attend, such as diabetics, wear a white paper tag indicating to volunteers that they should be served special diet ice cream and candy.

ICE CREAM BAR PROTECTORS. For picnics or parties, residents make a small slit in a paper plate which is slipped onto the sticks holding ice cream bars or fruit-sherbet lollipops. The paper plates catch the drips and help keep party clothes clean.

DRESSING IN COSTUME. At an infirmary patriotic parade, residents make Betsy Ross hats and kerchiefs for the ladies and cocked hats for the men. Leading the parade is a resident as a very impressive Uncle Sam; the color bearers give orders for marching, their oldest resident, ninety-nine, dressed in costume and seated in a decorated wheelchair. Twenty-three more wheelchairs follow with other residents in costume, holding flags and balloons, others beating drums or blowing horns. The dog mascot in the Home is decorated with a red, white, and blue ribbon bow, led by a resident and three clowns. Relatives watch and applaud.

PART III

SPECIAL PARTIES
AND
QUIZZES FOR ALL RESIDENTS

Chapter XIV

PARTIES FOR EVERY MONTH

COMPLETE PARTIES FOR RECREATION HALL GROUPS

One is always in danger of making the oldster feel that the activity is childish, that he is being insulted by a simple game, and fear of being laughed at may clinch his suspicions of being ridiculed.

One speaks to him as an equal, talks to him as a friend, gives him the chance to accept or reject the ideas — but the leader, and adult like himself he notices, seems to be having fun with it. In introducing the activity, the leader says, "This is like the game at the carnival," and shows him that it is. Or she says, "All men like to throw a ball; try it." Or, "Here's someone who needs a partner — give her a break."

If he still vehemently rejects it, she respects his decision but gives him a chance to change his mind. One ought not to mar his independence. If one of the party activities doesn't seem to be going well, one discards it or decides on a better time to try it but is sure to have something else to fall back on.

Not all of these activities will be suitable to every group and certainly not to every resident.

Newspaper Party (January)

Preparations: Newspapers, pins, scissors, Scotch tape, glue. With the aid of volunteers, residents make hats to wear during the party.

Newspaper Magic

While residents are busy doing this, five newspapers are arranged on the floor by the leader in the manner illustrated below.

263

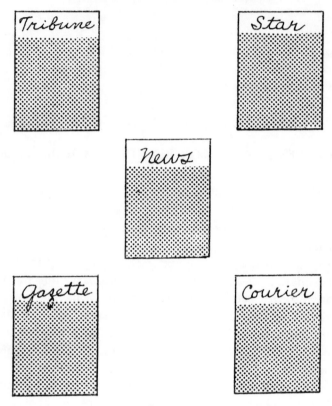

Fig. 36

Someone who has been told the secret of the stunt beforehand and has practiced sufficiently, is appointed by the leader as "it" and has left the room. The people in the room select a newspaper for him to guess. "It" must guess which newspaper the group has selected when he comes back into the room. The leader takes a long stick and may point to any paper saying "Is it this?", but the position of the stick on that first paper gives "it" the clue.

For instance, if number 1 were the paper chosen by the group, the leader would point to the upper left of any newspaper the first time he points, since the upper left corresponds to its position with the papers on the floor. Or if number 3 were chosen, the leader would point to the center of any newspaper when "it" first came into the room. After that, the leader could say,

"Is it this?" "Is it this?" pointing anywhere on any other papers in any order, since "it" knew the first time the leader pointed, which paper it was. The leader points to various papers and "it" continues to say "no" until the leader points to the correct newspaper. When other players think they know the solution, they may leave the room and try to guess.

Discovering the clue may take weeks and the game may continue as long as residents enjoy it.

Players may orally name as many words as they can get from the word "newspaper."

Newspaper Crime in Nursery Rhyme

You knew these when you were ten BUT do you know them now?

1. Who ran after the farmer's wife? (Three Blind Mice.)
2. Crime Section: Who stole a pig? (Tom the Piper.)
3. What crook walked with a crooked stick? (The Crooked Man.)
4. Who was one of the first girls to have real wolf trouble? (Red Riding Hood.)
5. Who killed all of his wives but one? (Blue Beard.)
6. What gal spent several nights in the woods with a company of little men? (Snow White.)
7. Lost and Found: Who lost some sheep? (Little Bo Peep.)
   Who lost some mittens? (Three Little Kittens.)

What's My Name?

One sentence at a time is read aloud by the leader; anyone in the circle raises his hand if he thinks he can identify the character. Five points could be given the first clue, four points on the next, three on the next, etc. When one runs out of descriptions, the residents make them up and try them on the group, perhaps including some obscure information about the superintendent or other employees. The most obscure statements come first in the description.

1. I gave my official salary to charities and to underpaid help. I was the thirty-first President, a Republican, born at West Branch, Iowa, in 1874. I got a degree in engineering and then became a mining engineer in Australia, Asia, Europe, Africa, and America. While in China, I directed food relief for people in the Boxer Rebellion. I became a world figure

in relief work. I distributed over five billion dollars' worth during 1914-1923. I was elected President over Alfred E. Smith. What's may names? (Hoover.)

2. I was born in Southampton, the daughter of a banker. I attended a private school and Vassar, studying the history of art at the Sorbonne one year. I was on the staff of the Washington **Times-Herald** and have been a farm worker and hospital volunteer. I became a camera fan. I speak French, Spanish, and Italian. I married in 1953. What's my name? (Jacqueline Kennedy.)

3. I am a flyer, an American stuntman, and a religious man. I was selected Father of the Year in 1962 by the National Father's Day Committee. I have two children. I am a lieutenant colonel; I am an astronaut made famous in 1962. What's my name? (John Glenn.)

4. I frequently make headlines all over the world. I cannot speak English, frequently lose my temper. I forcefully condemned the methods of Premier Stalin before the Soviet Communist party. I said Stalin led a cruel one-man rule that subverted the Communist aims. I was elected Premier in 1958, a position from which I was ousted. What's my name? (Krushchev.)

5. I have four children. I have a sister who married a photographer and who has one child. My father died in 1952, but my mother is still living. I receive from Parliament an annuity of over a million dollars a year, besides household expenses and salaries. My husband was the son of a Greek prince. I am the ruling sovereign of the House of Windsor. What's my name? (Elizabeth II.)

6. My children and husband, who was a lawyer, are now all deceased. I was born in Kentucky in 1818 and died 1882. My married life was stormy, and I was accused of undue extravagance in the White House. I was temporarily in a mental hospital. I was the daughter of Robert Smith Todd, a pioneer. What's my name? (Mary Todd Lincoln.)

7. I was born in Iowa but lived in Denver when I met my husband, a first lieutenant in the infantry at Fort Sam Houston.

Our first son died in infancy; our second is John, a graduate of West Point and a lieutenant colonel, married to Barbara Thompson. They have four children, Dwight David Eisenhower, II, Barbara Ann, Susan, and Mary Jean. What's my name? (Mamie Eisenhower.)

8. I'm a man in my forties — probably one of the most colorful figures of TV westerns. The men who work with me refer to me more often by my first name than my last. I took a character part, talked with a drawl, walked with a limp. What's my name? (Chester.)

9. I am a wealthy debutante from Main Line, Philadelphia. I've a fondness for slacks, English bicycles, left-wing literature, and modern art. Though my main interest is theater I made my first success as a warrior in a play and went clanging over the stage in armour. My first movie success was Jo in **Little Women.** I have red hair — really, I do — yes, really. What's my name? (Kathryn Hepburn.)

10. In my youth I was generally considered an ugly duckling. My chances of marriage didn't look so bright, so I took up social work. However I managed to make an excellent match. Although I was a mother and a grandmother, I was almost universally referred to by my first name. My most striking feature, I believe to be my teeth though I've never been sponsored by Pepsodent. In 1942 I visited troops in England. I had a weakness for travel and was seldom home. My friends tell me they were surprised to discover Winston Churchill had crossed the Rhine before I did. What was my name? (Eleanor Roosevelt.)

Leap Year Party (February)

(or Sadie Hawkins Party, November)

Decorations: Party decorations are left to the ingenuity of the committee. Turnabout ideas might be tried, such as chairs set backward and pictures faced against the wall. Simple decorations might be the silhouettes of the head of a man and woman, used to tack up on the walls or beds.

Introduction with a Kiss

Preparation: Molasses kisses.

Procedure: Each of the residents are passed molasses kisses and when everyone has his mouth filled, is asked to introduce himself. Volunteers may introduce themselves to the men as an ice breaker.

Mixers: Matching torn hearts, old sayings, or famous lovers, the volunteers look for their partners while the residents are seated. Another mixer might be spinning the bottle for partners with residents' names on slips arranged in a large circle on a table. Each volunteer spins a bottle and claims her partner as the name the bottle indicates.

Sleuthing

Preparation (items on the list given each couple):

The first beau (hair ribbon).

A drive through the wood (a nail partially driven into a small block of wood).

Hidden tears (onion).

Light of other days (candle).

A worn traveler (an old shoe).

Procedure: Working in pairs, volunteers hunt for the articles while residents give directions and write out the answers. Volunteers must not disclose the location of the articles, all in plain sight; as they discover them, they tell their partners, who write the answers.

Elopement

Preparation: Two of everything—umbrella, suitcase, large coat, and a woman's hat.

Procedure: Couples line up in two rows, each row with an umbrella and a suitcase in which are a large coat and a woman's hat. At a signal, the woman puts up the umbrella, picks up the suitcase, goes to the other end of the room, closes the umbrella, opens the suitcase, helps the man into the hat and coat, helps him take them off, puts them in the suitcase, picks up the closed umbrella and suitcase, and returns with her partner to hand things over to the next in line. This can be made as simple as necessary.

Taking the Match

Procedure: The leader reads the list and residents answer orally or, if this is too difficult, residents could be given slips from which to answer appropriately:

What clothes would a girl wear to land the following:

Scotsman? (Plaid.)	Fisherman? (Net.)
Musician? (Organdie.)	Banker? (Checks.)
Artist? (Canvas.)	Confectioner? (Taffeta.)
Barber? (Mohair.)	Milkman? (Jersey.)
Financier? (Cashmere.)	Gardner? (Lawn.)
Undertaker? (Crepe.)	Prisoner? (Stripes.)
Hunter? (Duck.)	Editor? (Prints.)

Beauty Contest

Preparation: Cold cream, mascara, eyebrow pencil, rouge, lipstick, powder, eye shadow.

Procedure: Allow each man to make up his partner as he thinks she should look from the arrangement on tables of the above beauty aids. Judges select winners. If there are enough couples competing, a grand march could be formed, the judges selecting the winning couple.

Refreshments: Wild cherry punch could be called love potion, the cookies, "honeymoon delight."

Serenade

Men sing songs about women and women sing songs with men's names, alternating until one team loses because it is not ready or because the song has been sung before.

Mardi Gras (February)

(including wards and recreation hall in the same activity)

Preparations: Costumes, masks for the residents to wear; refreshments; posters; wards may compete in decorations.

Procedure: Two resident-committee members are costumed and tour the Home bearing a sandwich board with announcement of the party. Handbills written and illustrated by bed patients can be distributed throughout the Home by two other costumed residents the day of the party.

Judging costumes, ward decorations, and picture taking can become the first part of the show.

MC may crown the king and queen of Mardi Gras.

A resident from the audience, blindfolded, is handed a set of women's apparel which he dons in view of the audience. If a suitable resident can't be found, an employee or volunteer who likes to clown will do.

The MC or a dancer from town might do a hula resplendent in a hula costume.

Heart Shuffle

Preparation: Four large paper hearts.

Procedure: Two residents compete. They place one foot on each paper heart, and they push the hearts down the aisle and back without losing them.

Heart Conundrums

Preparation: Any properties which would suggest the following:

Aspirin	Heartsick
Letters "AK"	Heartache
Weight	Heavy hearted
Torn paper heart	Broken hearted
Can of lye	Lion hearted
Stone	Heart of stone
Sugar	Sweetheart
Dripping red solution (fingernail polish)	Bleeding heart
Sponge	Soft hearted
Cut paper heart	Half hearted

Make up your own, too.

Contests: Guess how many cinnamon hearts in the jar; match pairs of lovers, etc.

Procedure: The audience guesses the answers.

Gay 90's Carnival (Valentine's Day) (February)

The "Kissing Booth"

Preparation: Bedside screens are set up to make a booth, over which are hung blankets or afghans to prevent anyone inside being seen; a raw potato is cut in two, the cut surface carved in the shape of lips; a lipstick.

Procedure: A barker "lures" men residents into the booth with much ballyhoo. Inside they are given their kiss with a potato, lipstick applied to the edge of a raw potato and stamped on the face of the oldster, who is asked not to reveal the secret of the booth.

The "Leg Toss"

Preparation: A girl and a rope ring.

Procedure: The girl sits on the table, and the men toss rope rings at her foot, the prize given for three tosses that are successful in succession.

Fortunes (auditorium activity).

Preparation: A cardboard circle in perhaps sixteen pie shapes, colored and labeled — biggest feet, happiest, biggest flirt, most handsome, biggest joker, has the heartiest laugh, biggest grin, biggest "line," most sentimental, most poetic, most shy, etc. An arrow pinned in the center is held at the back as the activity aide spins the card like a roulette wheel.

St. Patrick's Day Shenanigans (March)

Preparation: Darts, the map of Ireland; pennies, large paper shamrocks and St. Patrick's hats; card table covered with cigarettes, candy, apples, each in a separate pile; a pingpong net set up at the end, rope rings, cards; signs: "Danny's Den" and "Clancey's Corner"; fruit juice, cookies and coffee; green lapel tags and pins, a paper punch; a phonograph and Irish records.

Procedure: To report the score-keeping system, each resident is presented at the entrances with a green card on which he immediately writes his name. As he wins at any of the concessions, his card is punched. At the end of the afternoon cards are quickly and easily tallied to determine winners. Each game is run by an Irishman; and as the residents come in, each is given a shamrock with an assumed Irish name.

The games are the usual games dressed up in Irish clothing —

darts thrown at the map of Ireland, pennies pitched on shamrocks and St. Patrick's hats.

Another boon to any party could be a pin ball machine built
on a slant, with rubber sling shot to project the marbles up the
side of the board. A wheel of fortune indicates residents may
win either a bar of candy or gum or else they've had a run of
bad Irish luck.

As Irish sweepstakes continue throughout the afternoon, a
drawing is announced occasionally.

If the party committee feels that no St. Patrick's Day party
could possibly be complete without a bar, two can be set up
("Danny's Den" and "Clancey's Corner") with drinks named
"Mulligan's Mix," "Tom Collins," and "Mickey Finns," although
they are all the same fruit juice.

Hoop the Loot

Preparation: The card table is pushed against the wall, and
covered with cigarettes, candy and apples, each in a separate
pile; a pingpong net is set up at the end.

Procedure: The resident who stands or sits at the opposite end
of the table is given three rings to toss over the net. If he encir-
cles any article, it is his.

Paddy's Pig

Preparation: A square is roped off, the face of a large pig
drawn in the middle of the square and a horseshoe stake poked·
through his nose.

Procedure: Ringing the nose on Paddy's pig three times out of
five marks a winner.

Kiss the Blarney Stone

Preparation: A stone with a lovely girl's face painted or pasted
on the stone.

Procedure: One has to hold his right ankle with his left hand
while stooping over to kiss the lovely lips on the famous stone;
or he may be seated and the stone placed on the table.

Potato Tricks

Preparation: Potatoes and paring knives from the kitchen.

Procedure: Potato peeling contests for the longest unbroken peeling.

Pig Artistry

Preparation: Sheets of paper and pencil.

Procedure: Each "clan" is given a large sheet of paper and a pencil and as the leader calls the different parts of a pig the clan draws it with eyes closed; it is presented to the judges by the head of the clan, the clan receiving the winner's points.

Song Stunt

Procedure: Divided groups sing an Irish song at the same time, each singing a different song, one side, **"My Wild Irish Rose"** and the other, **"When Irish Eyes Are Smiling."** This can be carried out between two individuals rather than two groups.

Irish Sweepstakes

Preparation: Dice, play money, simple prizes.

Procedure: The following adaptation of the familiar horse race game illustrates a way of increasing resident participation. Human horses instead of the hobby horses can be used, the residents learning to run the program themselves.

Six lanes, each marked off by spaces on the floor, has six handicaps, saying "go back three spaces" or "six spaces," etc. Each space is numbered, and the "human horse" is given one dice which he shakes. He goes up the number of spaces on the dice; and if he is unlucky enough to land on one of the "handicap" spaces, has to go back the number directed. The residents mark the lanes on the floor and work out the handicaps ahead of time.

One resident worked out a betting system that does not even involve the handling of play money: As each resident enters, he is given a slip of paper containing a number. Before the start of each race, the residents come over, show their slips to the "bookie" and say, "I'm number eleven, and I'm betting on horse number four." The bookie has the numbers of each horse at the top of the page for each new race. Under each horse, he enters the numbers of the patients betting on that horse.

When the race is over, the residents on the winning horse collect their winnings, which are like bingo prizes — very small — three cigarettes, a stick of gum, etc. Each patient takes his turn at being a "horse."

Since all a "horse" has to do is to roll dice and move his chair up the required number of spaces, even wheeelchair residents become "horses." If at first it is difficult to get residents to move wheelchairs on the spaces, men on the committee may serve as the six horses.

Bit o' Blarney (March)

Decorations: Shamrocks, hats, pigs, and pipes; green and white crepe paper streams crisscross; curtains with shamrocks hung on them.

Preparation: A stone, any size; signs: "Kelly," "O'Toole," "McNamara," "Hooligan"; paper and pencils for all women present; four shillelaghs (sticks); record player or pianist with Irish music; crown or Irish hat; dime store novelty snake; eight corks, half of them blackened by being burned; list of Irish names, places, etc., to match the slips hidden in places in the room; four small tree branches; team prizes.

Procedure (pre-party activity): Guessing the weight of the Blarney Stone (any stone).

Procedure: Divide guests into four groups as Irish families and select Ma and Pa team leaders.

1. Kelly family.
2. O'Toole family.
3. McNamara family.
4. Hooligan family.

1. **Mixer.** "I've Got Your Number." Women get names of men residents in a given period of time. "Sleeper" — see how many of the residents noticed how many women had blue eyes.

2. **Pass the Shillelagh.** Each family forms a circle, and a shillelagh is passed as quickly as possible while an Irish record is played on the phonograph. When the music stops, the participant who has the shillelagh is out. Game ends when two people pass the shillelagh back and forth, and one ends up without the shillelagh.

3. **Selection of St. Patrick.** All the patients stand and are dropped out by responding to questions:
   (1) Everyone sit down that isn't at least one-half of one per cent Irish.

   (2) Everyone sit down who can't claim an Irish relative.

   (3) Everyone sit down whose grandparents (at least one) weren't born in Ireland.

   (4) Everyone sit down whose partner wasn't born in Ireland.

   (5) Everyone sit down who wasn't born in Ireland himself, etc.

   By process of elimination, "St. Pat" is selected, crowned with an Irish hat, and given a novelty snake for a prize.

5. **Irish Limerick or Toast to St. Pat.** Each "family" makes up a toast to St. Pat.

6. **Cork Game.** A man and woman face each other with small corks; only the woman's cork is burnt and makes marks on the man's face. Leader gives directions, and each partner gently rubs the other's face with the cork. The resident (or volunteer) ends up with a dirty face.

7. **Exhibition Irish Reel and Jig** if there are dancing residents.

8. **Sing Song.** Irish songs.

9. **Treasure Hunt for Shamrocks.** Each family is given a list of Irish names, places, etc., to find in the room. When each one is found, it's brought back and hung on the "family tree"; the team to finish first wins.

Refreshments are lime punch and ginger ale.

Easter Party (April)

(a party on the wards)

The Easter Decoration Contest

Decorations: All over the ward, bunnies peek from around corners; beautiful construction paper Easter eggs adorn walls, and everywhere Easter flowers, real and homemade, make their appearance in ward decorations made by the residents.

Preparation: Arrangements are made for an accordionist; residents distribute yellow paper chicks on which the program is written.

Procedure: The accordionist starts the party by going from door to door of the wards playing favorite melodies, followed by the activity aide and several residents rolling a medical cart piled high with equipment needed for the party. Each room is given a yellow chick with the program on it. After a brief explanation, the aide leaves necessary equipment in each room for the games and contests.

Miss Egg Face

Preparation: Sheets of large construction paper cut in an egg shape for each room.

Procedure: Patients in each room adorn a face on the large paper egg — pumpkin faces, pretty girls' faces, dog faces, etc.

Egg Guess

Preparation: Easter basket filled with bright colored paper eggs.

Procedure: Basket taken into each room; residents guess the correct number of eggs.

Selecting an Easter Parade Queen

Procedure: This can be developed in a number of ways; a week of nominations, campaign posters, PA speeches, closed ballot votes or a more simple afternoon activity of on-the-spot voting.

A more elaborate plan could be followed: A week before the party, preparations are made and wards notified about electing the Easter Parade queen. Names are submitted for each ward, residents and patients voting for five women; the winners are sent down the night of the party to compete with the five winners from each of the other wards. Each resident bed-patient lists the number of his choice from each ward; votes are counted and each ward queen selected and balloting held for the queen. A crown and fancy dressing gown are given her to wear and she has her picture taken with the king, whom she selects. Results are printed in the Home newspaper as well as the city paper.

Fashion Show

Preparation: Paper cups; plates; crepe paper; pins; feather and flowers; stapler, needles and thread; fine wire, and paste.

Procedure: Bed patients make hats from available material, and women residents model the hats in a fashion parade. Special hats are brought to the recreation hall or the front lobby and put on exhibit.

Spring Track Meet (May)

Potato Race

Preparation: Potatoes, toothpicks.

Procedure: Each contestant is given a toothpick and a potato. The potato must be rolled from start to finish line by continuous prodding with toothpicks on a long table.

Twenty-five Hurdle Race

Preparation: Obstacles such as boxes or chairs.

Procedure: Obstacles are placed over the designated distance contestants will take. Each contestant is assigned an assistant who will tell him where the obstructions are and how high or how low he or she must step to get over them. All contestants are given practice runs and are then assembled at the starting line and blindfolded. After this, obstacles are removed and the race begins, the assistants coached to walk along with them to protect them should they lose their balance.

Wheelbarrow Race

Preparation: Wheelbarrows are lined up.

Procedure: Contestants select partners and line up at starting line and push wheelbarrow to the finishing line and back (could be a wheelchair).

One-hundred-Yard Dash

Preparation: Each contestant has ten feet of string.

Procedure: One end of the string is attached to the small finger, the other to the fence (or anything similar). String must not be broken and must be coiled tightly around resident's hand; when the signal is given, he starts to wind.

Track Meet

Preparation: Cards, hats; dry cereal, spoons, blindfolds; needle threaders, thread; rolls of toilet paper; several match box covers; tissue paper disks and spoons; soft ball; coke bottles.

Procedure: **Shot-put** consists of tossing cards into hats; **twenty-five-yard dash,** blindfolded while feeding each other; **pole vault,** needle threading; the **half-mile,** cutting a roll of toilet paper down the middle without tearing; **the broad jump,** a relay in which men transfer a match box cover from nose to nose; **high jump,** another relay in which a tissue paper disk is carried on a spoon across the room and dropped into a box. The resident has a chance to earn extra points for his team by finding who has had the longest stay in the Home, the shortest time, is the tallest, or has the longest full name, etc. A **softball game** was played by swinging forward a ball which was suspended by a cord from the ceiling; the object of the game was to swing the ball forward and then on the return swing knock down a coke bottle.

Baseball Party (May)

Preparation: Suggested props would be pennants, crepe paper baseball caps, a baseball diamond drawn on wrapping paper or construction board, scoreboard, etc.

Procedure: Dividing residents into two teams, an equal number on each side, (an extra man may be used as an umpire) both ambulatory and nonambulatory may take part in the game. Each player has a baseball cap borrowed from a Little League team. Each team selects its own name and sets up a score board where everyone can see it.

Game No. 1 — Baseball Sports Quiz: A baseball diamond, 12″ by 12″, is drawn on poster paper and placed in a central position. Drawing pins are used as "runners" to mark bases and scores placed on the scoreboard at the end of each inning, the winning team given a pennant. The reader of the sports questions, is the umpire; a resident may be chosen. The batter answers the question and, if correct, goes to first base. If he fails to answer the question, he is out; and the umpire reads the correct answer and another question is asked of the next player. Questions have different values; for example, an easy question is a one-base hit; a more difficult question may by a two or three-base hit. The same team continues to bat until it has three outs. The game is called on account of rain or darkness when questions are depleted.

1. What is a pitch out? (Two-base hit.)
   Coach instructs pitcher to pitch to catcher who steps outside of catcher's box.

2. What is a squeeze play? (Two-base hit.)
   Runner is advanced from third to home by bunting.

3. What is a hit-and-run play? (Two-base hit.)
   Coach instructs batter to hit next ball and instructs base runner to start on the pitch.

4. What is the distance between bases? (One-base hit.)
   Ninety feet.

5. What is a bull pen? (One-base hit.)
   Place where pitchers warm up in front of the dugout.

6. How many warm up pitches are allowed a relief pitcher when he first comes in? (Three-base hit.)
   Six.

7. What is an assist? (Home run.)
   Player assisting a play by fielding the ball.

8. What is a triple play? (One-base hit.)
   Three outs made on the same play.

9. What is meant by a balk? (Home run.)
   Pitcher winds up, makes a definite motion to throw the ball over home plate and then throws elsewhere.

10. What is meant by a no hits, no runs, no errors game? (One-base hit.)

    Pitcher allows no hits or runs by the batter, and no errors are committed by the outfield.

11. If pitchers are changed during a game, which pitcher is credited with winning or losing the game? (One-base hit.)

    Essentially, the pitcher who is pitching when the winning run is scored.

12. What is meant by a triple? (One-base hit.)

    A three-base hit.

13. What is a double play? (One-base hit.)

    When two players on a team are put out at the same time.

14. What is an unassisted triple play? (Two-base hit.)

    When the fielder puts three men out on one play without the aid of his fellow players.

15. What is a hook slide? (Three-base hit.)

    Runner slides into base with one toe on the bag.

16. What is meant by a forced out? (One-base hit.)

    Runner is forced out by the runner behind him.

17. How many players on a baseball team? (One-base hit.)

    Nine.

18. When is a sacrifice hit made? (Two-base hit.)

    Batter bunts and is put out in an effort to advance runner.

19. What is a force play? (One-base hit.)

    If a batter hits fair, a runner on first base must go to second to make room for batter on first.

Game No. 2 — Dice Baseball: The same baseball diamond is used and play is called by use of a single die. Team No. 1 "bats," and each player gets one roll of the die. When team No. 1 has three "outs," No. 2 goes to "bat." The play is for nine innings and the count of the play is as follows:

1 — one-base hit	4 — home run
2 — two-base hit	5 — strike out
3 — three-base hit	6 — fly out

The winning team is given a pennant.

Baseball on Cards

Players: May be two individuals or teams.

Preparation: A deck of cards, chart of baseball diamond, and paper for scoring.

Procedure: The game can be played by two individuals who have baseball knowledge or, if desired, at a party where the group can be divided into three divisions — two teams and a spectator group. When team play is used, it is best to use a large wall chart of a baseball diamond and have players' names on cards that can be placed on the chart and moved as they proceed according to the rules of the game. Score should be kept on the chart, also outs and hits. This is advisable as it keeps the game visual and creates interest of both the players and the spectators.

The game works best when held to about five innings of play. If the five inning game is used and the interest is very high, a double header can be arranged. But a good recreation leader always arranges to have the game end when interest is still high for the best interest of future games.

Rules — One card is turned over at a time. When all cards are turned, shuffle and start over. All baseball rules of play are observed. The team at bat states, before the card is turned, whether the pitch is swung on or not.
The player says "out" when he intends to swing, "take" when he does not intend to swing at the ball. Three out is an inning.

Errors — When a Joker is cut, runners can advance one base; batter goes to first.

Stealing — The intention of stealing must be announced. If successful, the runner advances one base. Even cards make the steal safe, odd cards, an out.

Double Steal — Intention must be announced. Two even cards make a successful double steal.

Other — All advances on passes, wild throws and pick offs can be card combinations, if players wish to be very technical.

Card Values and Symbols — These may look complicated but are easily learned. Note that spades and hearts have the same value as diamonds and clubs.

SPADES OR HEARTS

Cut	Take
Ace — Out	Ball
King — Single, runner advances two bases	Ball
Queen — Fly out, no advance	Ball
Jack — Fly out, no advance	Ball
Ten — Out	Ball
Nine — Fly ball, advance one base	Base
Eight — Fly out, no advance	Ball
Seven — Fly out, advance one base	Ball
Six — Fly out, advance one base	Ball
Five — Out	Ball
Four — Fly out, advance if man on third	Ball
Three — Fly out, advance one base	Ball
Two — Double play if man on. If not, one out	Ball

DIAMONDS OR CLUBS

Cut	Take
Ace — Home Run	Strike
King — Single, if man on, advance two bases	Strike
Queen — Fly out, no advance	Strike
Jack — Double-runner, advance two bases	Strike
Ten — Strike out	Strike
Nine — Fly out, no advance	Strike
Eight — Fly out, no advance	Strike
Seven — Single, runner advances one base	Strike
Six — Fly out, runner on advances one base	Strike
Five — Triple	Strike
Four — Fly out, man advance only if on third	Strike
Three — Fly out, advance one base	Strike
Two — Double play if man on base. If not, one out	Strike

Triple Play — If there are two or three runners on base and the batter turns over a two on a cut which constitutes a double play, the opposition may demand that the batter pick another card. If this card is a three of any suit, it becomes a triple play.

Summer Carnival (June)

Decorations: Each committee is responsible for a concession. Posters are made on wrapping paper with large letters announcing contents of the booth, or wrapping paper around the legs of a card table announcing the concession. The tent is plastered with large wrapping paper signs and also large pictures of "characters" at the end of the tent where photographer is stationed.

Preparations: Properties needed are a barker with megaphone, envelopes with paper money counted out previously and a supply of paper money at each concession to make change; prizes; turtles and a paper racetrack marking the distance to their run; bingo; dolls or animals and ball; freaks and wonders prepared ahead of time; artist and art material for sketches, or photographer and camera, and money to make change; snake show previously prepared; the black cardboard box in the shape of a camera and the black cloth, which could be used for the man posing as photographer who climbs for an "angle"; a chair for the customers and the magazine character pictures previously mounted to give away.

Tin Can Alley

Preparation: Six to ten cans with faces painted on them; three soft balls; one red large table; two screens used as background or some sort of backstop.

Decorations: Varicolored flags outlining booth; sign giving the odds.

Procedure: Player is given three chances to knock all cans off the table; cans stacked three — two — one.

Silhouette Booth (*Must be in a closet or dark room.*)

Decorations: Silhouettes of employees.

Preparation: One goose neck lamp with strong bulb (100 watt); supply of large sheets of dark colored paper (12" x 18") — black is best for silhouettes; supply of white or pastel paper, same size on which to mount silhouettes; stapling machine to attach picture to mounting; a soft lead pencil; a pair of scissors.

Procedure: 1. Lamp is on a level with the subject's head and set about 8′ away. Leader experiments with the angle of the light to get a clear profile shadow on the wall. 2. Subject is seated with shoulder against wall to prevent sway. 3. Image is traced profile on dark paper and cut out. Slight changes can be made for beauty's sake, e.g., necks slimmed, etc. 4. Silhouettes mounted on white paper.

Shooting Gallery

Preparation: Two guns, four rounds of ammunition for each gun (the rubber suction cups), two targets and prizes. The targets are nailed to a tree and then the booth set up, using streamers and pennants. The targets are metal trays on which the suction cups will stick — warm water and glycerin help — and rings painted on the targets, 20, 30, and 50 (bull's eye).

Procedure: The contestant stands eight feet away from the target and he gets four shots at the target. If he hits the bull's eye or makes 80 points, he wins a prize. Two volunteers help run it.

Pitching Booths

Preparation: Hoop of wire, five paper plates. Large picture of a nurse on cardboard, the eyes and mouth especially prominent; a sign above the picture reads "Wink Her Eye or Smack Her Lips and Win a Prize"; a large table.

1. Pitch Woo to the Nurse

Procedure: The contestants are given five pennies to toss from a specified distance; if one lands directly on the eyes or mouth, he is awarded a prize. A large table is needed upon which the picture is laid nearly flat.

2. Pie Pitching

Preparation: A large hoop of wire is suspended at a height of eight feet.

Procedure: The contestant stands approximately five feet in front of the wire hoop and is given five paper plates to toss through the hoop, two out of five entitling him to a prize.

Pinata

Preparation: This Mexican idea for special parties such as at Christmas, birthdays, and carnivals is a large heavy paper sack or cardboard box used as a container (in Mexico a pottery vase is used) filled with wrapped candy (candy kisses or mints), peanuts and some fruit, the outside decorated with many colors of crepe paper or tissue with many streamers. It may be a fancy box type or it may represent a figure, a bird or a basket of flowers, with elaborate decorations, such as a witch for Halloween and a Santa Claus at Christmas time.

Procedure: The piñata is hung from the ceiling with a cord extending through a hook at each side of the ceiling, with two people holding each end to lower or raise the piñata avoiding the residents' blows in striking it. The guests, who each in turn are given a stick and blindfolded, try three times to break the piñata. The rope swings away with the resident finally breaking the container, and the "goodies" are scattered.

All residents keep a distance from the piñata as to avoid getting hit by the bat or stick. The blindfolded resident holds tightly to the bat, so it does not slip out of his hand as he swings.

July Carnival

Publicity: One can use all the discarded strings of flags from the local filling station.

Large attractive posters advertising the carnival date, time and place are put up on the bulletin boards in the Home, announcements made on the PA. On the day of the carnival, residents dress in costumes or paper hats, flying balloons, beating drums, and carrying sandwich signs go through the dining room at dinner time.

Preparation: Peep Show: Several bridge tables gayly decorated with streamers, flags, balloons, etc., are placed in a row.

Cigar boxes painted different colors are placed on the tables. Signs, like the ones given below are placed on them and they will actually contain the corresponding properties.

Signs:	Properties:
The hairless dog	Hot dog
Undressed kid	Kid glove
Remains of ancient Greece	Candle
Black bottom	Bottom of skillet

Procedure: Pegs are driven in the ground and paper strung from one to the next so that spectators walk in a line to view the show rather than gather in groups.

Beat Your Number Gambling Game

Preparation: Card table (covered with brown paper field) on which squares are numbered one to eighteen; four checkers, three dice.

Procedure: Player puts checker on the number he wishes to make. He has five chances to get that number as the total on the three dice.

Planning, serving and preparation of drinks or food may be necessary. A volunteer attends each concession, running errands, keeping supplies going, operating with the help of the resident committee in charge.

Procedure: A barker, a man with a megaphone or loud speaker at the entrance of the tent, announces the wonders; residents sitting at entrance take tickets from customers.

Everyone is given an envelope containing the same amount of paper money to use as he likes. At the end of the afternoon he's given a prize, depending on how much money he has won.

Turtle Race. Real dime store turtles each containing a name or number on the back run a race; a bookie takes the play money, starts the turtles off, announces the winners and makes the payoffs.

Freaks and Wonders of the World. A bearded lady (wearing a false beard or mustache); man with the pointed head (man wearing a point stuck on with "nutty putty" or spirit gum); frog man (wearing rubber flippers on his feet); fat man or lady (wearing pillow padding); Mr. Schnozzle (with false nose); Seven Seas (a box with a peek hole and 7C's); World's Most Horrible Monster (a mirror); Flying Saucer (fly in saucer); Boxing Matches (box of matches); Ruins of China (broken dish); Original Comb and Brush Set (twig from a tree); Unusual Lead Formation (lead pencil); For Women Only (hair pins); For Men Only (cigar). Residents pay paper money to see the shows.

Sketch Artist. A photographer takes pictures with a polaroid camera for residents willing to pay for the cost of the film.

Snake Show. Shoe boxes are decorated with a peek hole at the top of the boxes and signs labeling them "Rattler" (with a baby rattle inside); "Garter" (a lady's garter); "Diamond" (a dime store ring); "Copperhead" (a penny); "Pine Snake" (pine cone or needles); "Moccasin Snake" (a moccasin); "Grass Snake" (grass).

Photographer. The resident poses in a chair with a formal setting rigged up with a backdrop. The volunteer pretends to be taking a picture of the person posing, disappearing back of a box, his head and the box covered with a large black cloth. She gives the resident a picture cut from a magazine mounted on a cardboard: a beautiful young girl, a celebrity, or anything this resident will think is funny.

Weight Guessing. Someone tries guessing a resident's weight and then puts the resident on the scales to verify the weight. If he is off by ten pounds, the resident is given a prize or the paper money. Age could also be guessed if residents like this idea.

Fiesta (August)

Decorations: Posters:

Hagame usted el favor
Senorita and Senor
De venir a nuestra Fiesta
Won't you come to our gala Fiesta?

Mexican Fiesta. Scene: infirmary patio with tables set-up for cabaret with "puestos" around the edge of the hall or lawn. Crepe paper festoons, fringed tissue paper eight inches wide of many gay colors . . . flowers everywhere and plants to suggest a garden, clusters of fruit (painted) or big balloons of various sizes to look like fruit. Cactus plants, Mexican scenes with burros, pottery, hats, birds, parrots, and macaws. The festoons or fringed paper can form a canopy either for inside or outdoors.

Tables, carts, and booths or "puestos" are gaily decorated with bright colored paper.

Preparations: Puestors — These are booths arranged around the hall with colorful signs — "refrescos" for the pop or punch stand . . . "comedas" for the food served such as popcorn, peanuts in shell, Fritos®, candy, and cookies . . . Several puestos for contests such as "jumping beans," "frijole pitch," "bala," and "los caballos."

Musica — A music stand or stage setup with a Mexican orchestra, marimba, and group of singers in costumes with all Spanish music or records.

Hostesses — A group of hostesses or college girls may come in gay Spanish costumes or bright full skirts and blouses, with flowers in their hair.

Jumping Beans

Procedure: Residents bet on the bean to jump out of circle first, tickets given to each winner.

Frijole Pitch

Preparation: Container filled with water with a small glass jar in center.

Procedure: Each one tries to toss five Mexican beans into the jar, tickets given to any resident getting all five beans in the jar.

Bola

Preparation: This is a "tenpins" type of game. Spanish use only three bowling pins, set in a row in front of player. Center pin counts twelve points and others six points.

Procedure: Two residents bowl at a time and highest score gets the ticket.

Los Caballos

Preparation: Six numbered horses from chess set and checkerboard.

Procedure: Each resident chooses horse, using dice for moves on checkerboard; winner also receives ticket.

The individual holding most tickets at end of evening receives a prize. Gay music of some sort as a background for the Fiesta all evening adds to atmosphere.

Making Sombreros

Preparation: An assortment of oval shaped cardboards or heavy paper, cut the size of the top of a hat, and the same materials cut into brims; scissors and paste or Scotch tape.

Procedure: Perhaps with the assistance of a volunteer, residents assemble the hats and wear them.

Cock Fight

Preparation: Colorful drawings of four roosters in a fighting position, red, green, blue, and yellow — are a means of dividing group into teams; small cocks are pinned on each, or just a tag of color to designate team they're on. Fringed paper in four colors, which represent feathers, are hidden around the room.

Procedure: All hunt as a team to find their feathers and paste on bird; the most attractively finished cock receives the point for their side.

Do You Know Your Spanish?

Procedure: This contest is like a spelling bee. Two members from each team are chosen; one gets a chance at a question. If he misses, a member of the other team gets a try at it. Spanish words or phrases are used until one team is a winner. Define: peso, Mexican dollar; frijole, bean; charro, cowboy; agua, water; hacienda, ranch; patio, outdoor courtyard; serape, blanket; rio, river; colorado, red; sombrero, hat; piñata, a decorated container filled with goodies; hasta mañana, until tomorrow; hasta la vista, until we meet again; viva la, long live.

"Charro" Round Up

Preparation: Four sombreros, four canes, and two small milk bottles, decorated to look like a small steer by pasting a steer head on neck of bottle, perhaps.

Procedure: There are two contestants from each team, each given a sombrero, cane, and a small milk bottle between them. The four contestants, "caballeros," mount their "horses" and at a given signal begin to round up their steer into the corral. At this point each "charro" waiting at corral changes places with first "charro" taking sombrero and stick and mounting "caballo," the wooden horse. The object is to see who can get his steer back to home corral first, since the bottle will whirl and zigzag on the floor.

School Day Party (September)

Preparation: Record player, variety of records sung in foreign tongue, whatever is available; three or four sheets of paper and pencil for each one present; blackboard or large sheet of butcher's paper taped on the wall for drawing. States cut out, unidentified and numbered on the wall; large county or state map outline.

A few curved lines drawn on sheets of paper to be distributed as "doodles" to which the residents may add any lines or drawings which may result in simple "arty," "interesting," or realistic drawings for their evaluation or amusement.

Decorations: Imitation of old-fashioned slate with a childish scrawl and names of residents to stay after school; maps, cutouts, school pennants on walls; teacher's desk. Teacher dressed severely, wearing glasses.

Procedure: Opening. All sing "School Days."

Music Appreciation: Identify language in foreign songs.

Third Class: Geography (orally)

1. Geography quiz. (Residents answer with abbreviation of states.)
   a. What state is a girl's name? Minn.
   b. What state is a Catholic church service? Mass.
   c. What is Noah's state? Ark.
   d. What state is a physician? Md.
   e. What state is a mineral substance containing metal? Ore.
   f. What state is a personal pronoun? Me.
   g. What state suggests Monday? Wash.
2. Residents identify states by outlines, unidentified state outlines, numbered on a wall.
3. Residents put an "X" on home location on a county map, or the place of birth on a state map.

Spelldown

Spell these words backwards:

1. Books — skoob.
2. Paper — repap.
3. Chalk — klahc.
4. Grade — edarg.
5. Pupil — lipup.
6. Write — etirw.
7. Dunce — ecnud.

First Class: Arithmetic (written)

1. Each resident writes his age and month of birthday. For October (10th month), age 50 he writes:

Number of the month	10
Multiply by 2	20
Add 5	25
Multiply by 50	1250
Add his age	1300
Subtract 365	935
Add 115	1050

2. Farmer's Plot (Written). A farmer has four sons and wants to divide his farm into four equal plots, each the same size and shape. Can they divide it for him?

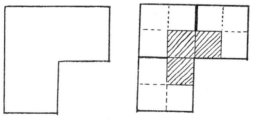

Fig. 37

3. Residents with aid of pencil and paper, add these figures; first one to finish is the winner. Add 75, 35, 47, 53, 64, 76, 90, 50, 10. Answer, 500.

Second Class: English

1. He answers these questions orally:
    a. If a boy ate his father and mother, what would he be?
       Orphan.
    b. How do you spell "blind pig?" Pig without an eye.
    c. What is the longest sentence in the world? Life.
    d. Make one word out of "new door." One word.

Spirit Spree (October)

Decorations: Eight tables set up with chairs and standards
on tables display symbols for eight teams (jack o'lantern, witch,
cat, bat, ghost, goblin, skeleton, and scarecrow). Cutouts of
witches, bats, etc., on walls in recreation hall, on refreshment
table, and on stage curtains. Two residents go through wards
with sandwich sign, "Which Witch Has the Toni?" on front, and
party information on back.

Preparation: Blackboard for scoring; felt scraps, yarn, feathers,
ribbon; eight pumpkins, eight knives; eight oranges; eight apples
on strings; pianist, blackboard with scrambled "Halloween" word;
MC; doughnuts and cider.

Jack O'Lantern Carving Contest
Procedure:

The group of residents form competing teams. Each team is
given a pumpkin and a knife to cut a jack o' lantern (using other
scrap material to decorate). There is a twenty minute time limit;
judges are representatives from each team. Apples are hung on
string from peg board or curtains on stage. First contestant
finishing hanging five apples gets twenty-five points; second,
twenty points; all others ten points.

Trick or Treat

A volunteer MC shows each team a scrambled "Halloween"
word on blackboard. Team must answer before MC counts to
five, or do a trick.

Scrambled Words

Words could be boglin (goblin); tichwes (witches); carescrow (scarecrow); muppkin (pumpkin); tootkcsirbm (broomstick); bgabblepoping (apple bobbing); batclack (black cat), and loonmight (moonlight).

If correct answer is given, ten points are awarded. Each team which does not get word in allotted time must do the "trick." Four men from the team pass an orange under their chins from one person to another using no hands. Team which finishes first gets twenty-five points; second, twenty points; other contestants, ten points each. This activity takes place on stage or where all residents can watch activities and cheer their team.

Spirit of Song

This time the MC reads a question, and pianist plays answer. Team which calls out the song title first gets five points for each correct answer. Questions and answers follow, but any other suitable songs are acceptable.

1. When Johnny asked "Trick or Treat" and didn't get a treat, what did he yell? **"Who Threw the Overalls in Mrs. Murphy's Chowder?"**

2. What question might you ask of yourself when you saw a group of ghosts on Halloween? **"Did You Ever See a Dream Walking?"**

3. What is the best weather forecast we could make to ward off the spirits on Halloween? **"Ain't Going to Rain No More."**

4. When do the pranksters start to make their rounds on Halloween? **"In the Gloaming."**

5. In what are the witches very busy making brew on Halloween? **"Little Brown Jug."**

6. What do you see by the light of on Halloween? **"Harvest Moon."**

7. What did the goblin say to the witch he met on Halloween? **"I Love You Truly."**

8. What usually happens on a Halloween night? **"There'll Be a Hot Time in the Old Town Tonight."**

9. When would you overtake a platoon of goblins on Halloween night bouncing? **"By the Light of the Silvery Moon."**

10. What do you say to a ghost on a dark road on Halloween? **"I'm Looking over a Four Leaf Clover."**

11. What do you duck for on Halloween? **"Don't Sit under the Apple Tree."**

12. Where's the favorite hangout for the ghost on Halloween? **"Down by the Old Mill Stream."**

13. If you walked by a graveyard on Halloween night, what song might you hear? **"Hail, Hail, the Gang's All Here."**

14. What did Johnny say to Sammy while they were discussing their plans for Halloween night? **"Our Boys Will Shine Tonight."**

15. What did Susie cry out as she met a goblin on Halloween? **"Show Me the Way to Go Home."**

16. What did the witch say about how she felt as she climbed aboard her broomstick? **"I'm Sitting on Top of the World."**

17. What sounds did Johnny hear in the haunted house that made him run home? **"Tramp, Tramp, Tramp."**

18. What does everyone hope to have a little bit of on Halloween night? **"With a Little Bit of Luck."**

Superstitions

Flash cards with a picture suggesting a superstition to the teams. The team which recognizes the superstition connected with each and calls out correct answer, gets five points (black cat, walking under a ladder, number 13, etc.)

Ghost Stories

This activity is used if time permits. Each team is given a slip of paper with the following beginning of a story: "It was on a black, gloomy night as we were walking down the lonely lane when . . . ." A ten minute time limit is given. At the conclusion, a representative from each team stands on the darkened stage and reads the ghost stories composed by his "team." By applause, points are given: first place, twenty-five; second, twenty; all others, ten.

Running scores are kept of teams scoring, team accumulating the most points served first for refreshments.

Spin the Bottle

Procedure: After the leader finds who wants their fortune told, he spins the bottle and reads the fortune from the cards where the bottle points.

Fortunes for Spin the Bottle

1. The best way to liven up a party may be for you to leave.
2. The trouble with life is, you're half way through before you realize it's one of those "do-it-yourself deals."
3. Minds are like parachutes, no good unless opened.
4. It's smart to pick your friends, but not to pieces.
5. The man in the moon isn't half so interesting as a lady in the sun.
6. You shift your brain into neutral and let it idle on.
7. Few of us get dizzy from doing too many good turns.
8. You are God's gift to the squirrels.
9. A handful of patience is worth more than a bucket full of brains.
10. Christmas greetings speak of peace on earth — but they don't say where.
11. Let the girls go on their way; for you they need not stay.
12. Rich food and late hours are what make a lot of people thick and thin.
13. An escaped leopard is believed to be spotted.
14. It's not what you do, it's what you get away with.
15. No matter how it's sliced, it's still bologna.
16. If you think you're too old for growing pains, try spading a garden.
17. If it's a small world, why does it cost so much to run it?
18. When a woman suffers in silence, it means her phone is out of order.
19. Give some people an inch, and they think they're rulers.
20. Don't look into a mirror; you might break it.
21. There are bigger things in life than money — bills.
22. The happiest miser on earth is one who saves friends.
23. The grass next door may be a bit greener, but it's just as hard to cut.

24. You have a heart like a trolley car — always room for one more.

25. Middle age is when your waist and broad mind begin to change places.

26. There may not be much to see in a small town, but what **you do** see makes up for it.

27. Hard work is the yeast that raises the dough.

28. You are as fresh as a new laid egg.

29. Conceit is a strange disease; it makes everyone sick except the one who has it.

30. The first place to look for a helping hand is at the end of your arm.

31. A replacement for TV's late show — it's called SLEEP.

32. You are the apple of my eye.

33. Don't be like a fence — running around a lot without getting anywhere.

34. Don't go looking for the ideal man; a husband is much easier to find.

35. When you slide down the banister of life, we hope the splinters are facing the same way.

36. The only way to save money nowadays is to have short arms and deep pockets.

37. You'll never get into trouble by talking.

38. You are a genius in disguise.

39. If you want to forget all your troubles, wear tight shoes.

40. You are such a good gardener that all that comes up is your water bill.

41. You love to sing and dance and play and flirt the livelong day.

42. All you need is a hook; you have a good line.

43. You are much too smart for your breeches.

44. Some cars have fluid drive; others just have a drip at the wheel.

Football Party (November)

Preparation: Footballs cut out of paper and hidden around the room; paper bags; beanbags and chairs; football quiz, balloons; refreshments of popcorn and punch; phonograph and college song records.

Procedure: Captains are chosen who help make up cheers or slogans.

1. Kickoff and captains flip coins to start.

    First Quarter: Find the football: teams search for pieces of their football hidden around the room and piece them together. Point after touchdown: paper bag relay; six men from each team line up. Each man in turn goes to a chair and picks up a paper bag, blows it up and breaks it, then goes back to his team.

    Second Quarter: Point after touchdown: Sir Walter relay; one player stands in front of the other player and moves the pieces of paper on which he stands so the player can move forward. When they get to the end, the players exchange places.

    Third Quarter: Point after touchdown: falling on the ball; beanbag is placed on a chair; and teams are lined up and numbered. When the leader calls on a number, the two men with that number try to get the bag back to his line without being tagged. Two points if he succeeds, are scored.

    Fourth Quarter: Football quiz (can be on anything). Each team gets a chance to answer a question if he catches the football. Point after touchdown: interference relay; six couples from each side are chosen. Around the ankle of each volunteer is fastened a balloon; the couples link arms and the men try to break the other balloons while protecting their own.

Refreshments of popcorn and punch are served while scores are counted and phonograph plays college songs.

Touchdown Time

Procedure: Captains of each team choose, and coin is flipped to see which team begins with ball in their possession. There are questions on cards from one to sixty-one, with yardage gained on each. Each team has four questions to answer (downs). If all four are answered, the team is able to continue for four more questions. If a team cannot answer the question, the other team is able to try and answer it. If the opponents answer correctly, they receive the ball and the yardage (intercepted pass). Play is begun on the fifty-yard-line at the beginning of the game and after each touchdown. The team must be able to get over their goal line for a touchdown. After a touchdown is made, the team answers another question.

Round-up Party (November)

Decorations: Construction paper, pencils, scissors, and patterns for decorations, used by the residents tracing and cutting out cacti, bucking broncos, ranch brands, mounting cutouts on posts and stage curtains; brown butcher paper will simulate fencing. Publicity perhaps consists of posters, a notice in the Home newspaper, and by "word of mouth" through the residents' council and PA system.

Preparation: Ten teenage hostesses, card tables with materials for making paper neckties of various colors of crepe paper and scissors.

Procedure: When the teenage hostesses arrive, the aide meets them and explains the party; the girls are asked to help with the activities and mix with the residents.

With the help of some of the residents, volunteers make western neckties which are pinned on the residents after they come in. Card tables are placed on the sides of the room and decorated appropriately.

Booth: Rope of the Muley Cow

Preparation: A large cardboard cow's head is mounted on a broom, perhaps tied to a microphone stand, placed between stage curtains, or placed back of a plywood "corral"; a rope lasso.

Procedure: Residents stand or sit in wheelchairs within marked boundary and attempt to lasso her in five tries.

Jack Rabbit Shot

Preparation: Four jack rabbits cut out of stiff cardboard (left from Easter) are fastened on individual stands, each about four-teen inches high, painted a different color and placed on a high shelf (perhaps the top of a coat rack stand) where they can be knocked off easily.

Procedure:

Each resident is given four tennis balls and tries to knock down all four rabbits at a distance of about ten feet.

Two teenagers can run this concession, one to set up the rabbits and one for a barker to give out the balls and points.

Wild Animal Pistol Range

Preparation: Pictures of cardboard animals lined along a shelf, for a rifle range; toy rifle.

Procedure: Toy rifles with cork bullets are used to shoot the animals down.

Party Activities: Human Scavenger Hunt

Preparations: While briefing them and explaining the party to the hostesses, slips of paper are given to each; the hostesses are to get as many signatures as possible from the residents who have done something unusual. They try to find out by talking with them who has had the most cows to milk, who has had the biggest family, farmed the longest time, has the most children who are farmers, had the most unusual farm, etc.

Chit Chat Circle

Preparation: Music.

Procedure: (This is for ambulatory residents.) Arranged in the order of a mixer, residents form an outside circle and teen-agers, an inside circle.) On a signal, both circles rotate in oppo-site directions. When the music stops, people opposite each other converse for one minute on a given topic: why I like my town, my favorite dinner, the holiday (whatever is nearest) I like best, my favorite time of year, etc.

The activity can end with a grand march formed by dissolving the two circles into one huge circle. One couple chosen as head couple leads the others down the middle of the recreation hall in pairs of twos, one pair going one way, the next pair the other way. The pairs circle the room and then meet to form groups of four, then eights. After forming groups of eights, the units split into pairs again, forming arches through which everyone behind them must go and then they form arches too. When all arches have been formed, the head couple goes through the line of arches with the next couple following, finally dissolving the arches and forming a great circle. The grand march, done to music, proves a fitting climax to the Chit Chat Circle.

White Elephant Party (December)

Preparations: This is good for that "letdown week after Christmas." Volunteers collect the wrapped packages in a white elephant box contributed by residents and volunteers, after an announcement such as this: "After the holidays, we think of 'white elephants,' things which we have received that we do not need and might like to get rid of. Each of you will be given ribbon, paper, and a used Chistmas card. Take something you don't want from your bedside table or wallet and wrap it. Your white elephant gift will be collected in the white elephant box and distributed to some lucky fellow or lady later on."

White elephant and pink elephant cutouts are distributed to all patients. This party is chiefly planned as a hostess or volunteer-directed party adapted to a bedridden ward or may be adjusted to a general party of semi-ambulatory residents. Decorations, while not planned for this party, would be helpful but not necessary.

Procedure: Half the ward is given small white elephants, half pink elephants; and everyone is given a quiz sheet. Team is given fifteen points which has the most patients scoring fifteen correct answers or more.

Elephant Flip

Procedure: On one tray are placed eleven white elephants numbered from two to twelve and a pair of dice; on the other tray, eleven pink elephants and dice. Object of the game is to turn all elephants face down. The patient rolls the two dice. If he rolls an eight, he turns down the number eight elephant or a combination of elephants totaling eight. He may roll the dice until he rolls a number for which there is no single elephant nor combination of elephants left to turn down. He totals the numbers of the elephants left, face up. Low scorer on each team wins a bag of peanuts or some prize.

After totaling team scores, the volunteer passes white elephant box to winning team, first letting them choose their white elephant package.

White Elephant Phrases

(Worn out ones, that is; residents can complete them.)

Phrases	Answers
1. I just washed my hair . . .	(1) and I can't do a thing with it.
2. New York is a fine place to visit but . . .	(2) I'd hate to live there.
3. He comes from a poor but . . .	(3) honest family.
4. It's not the heat, it's . . .	(4) the humidity.
5. Pardon me, but . . .	(5) your slip is showing.
6. Unaccustomed as I am . . .	(6) to public speaking.
7. How long are you going to be in that . . .	(7) bathroom.
8. It's not what she says . . .	(8) it's the way she says it.
9. It was so foggy, you . . .	(9) couldn't see your hand in front of your face.
10. She's old enough to be . . .	(10) his mother.
11. It's not the company, it's . . .	(11) the hour.
12. Never say . . .	(12) "die."
13. What was good enough for my mother . . .	(13) is good enough for me.
14. When you say that, brother . . .	(14) smile.
15. If I've told him once . . .	(15) I've told him a hundred times.
16. The truth . . .	(16) hurts.
17. I like to see young people . . .	(17) enjoy themselves.
18. Stop me if you've . . .	(18) heard this before.
19. Can you lend me five . . .	(19) till payday?
20. The best things in life are . . .	(20) free.

SPECIAL PARTY PROGRAMS

All States Party

Preparation: Lapel markers for everyone; names of towns on slips, a large map of the state, blindfolds.

Procedure: Each resident is given a lapel marker of his home town when he arrives. Each resident draws the name of a town from a basket, then without disclosing the name, describes it, gives an opinion, anecdote or story, while the others guess what town is under discussion.

"Airplane" is a game using a large map of the state or county placed at one end of the room; the contestant walks blindfolded across the room pinning his lapel name tag on his home town; if he arrives in his home town, he has made a nonstop airplane flight home.

Sports Party

Sportsmen's Stag Party or Smoker

First of all, a good date must be chosen. When there is to be, or has been, some sports event of great interest, the residents' interest is greater. Besides an awareness of sports one must also have an attraction to draw the residents to the party. If this is to be stag and no women present, the attraction has to be very persuasive. It would be great to have someone like Stan Musial or Jack Dempsey come to the affair; but since this is probably impractical, the next best thing is the sports writer for the local paper or radio or TV sports announcer, or a man from the State Conservation Department, a high school coach, or football captain. There's bound to be someone around who knows about sports and who could be persuaded to lend his support to a worthy cause. Now that the interest has been created and the guest persuaded, the environment is next.

Preparation: A sports event of interest to the residents is announced and residents prepare some questions for discussion with the guest speaker. Residents might meet in a group circle on the ward, or move their beds out in the solarium, if that's possible.

Sports events, news and pictures, can be put on the bulletin board illustrating golf, fly-tying, high school basketball — whatever is likely to interest them most.

Residents might work up a sports scrapbook of their individual interest; the scrapbook could then be kept in the lounge for other residents to read. If residents have any sport trophies, they might bring them to show the guest. A big poster on the wall with pictures of famous sports figures makes the event interesting; pictures of sportsmen can be cut up and mixed up so that Babe Ruth's head might be on Jack Dempsey's body or placed on the neck of a movie star, for instance.

Record player and the record, "Great Moments in Sports": the record should be studied beforehand and an outline of questions made.

Procedure: Residents are asked to identify the famous sports figures on the wall. When the guest arrives, he might take part, to become acquainted with the residents. As participants finish and gather in a circle, the guest is introduced and gives a short talk on his specialty or any important sports event he cares to talk about on an informal basis; the residents are free to ask questions as they like.

If the question and discussions seem to roll along with no need for a change, continue; but if questions seem forced or there are periods of silence, it is best to start something else. The winner of the "Famous Figures" is announced or the record, "Great Moments in Sports" may be played for residents to identify many famous voices or events, with perhaps the guest speaker starting; each person present could give his favorite sports memory or tall fish story.

Activities will depend entirely on questions and discussions brought about by the speaker and participants. If the group is at ease and enjoying themselves, it could very well continue until refreshments are served. Other activities could be started with the guest taking part if he is able to stay. The following quizzes could be used, if the need arises, done orally, calling out questions and soliciting the answers with no competition involved:

Gone Fishing!!!

1. Do flying fish have wings?   No.
2. The fishing reel is a development of the nineteenth century! True........ False (F).
3. About what percentage of Americans would you say engage in the sport of fishing?   Twenty per cent.
4. Records prove that fishermen are primarily interested in finding a "good fighting fish."   True .... False (F).
5. Do fishermen and hunters spend more money for licenses or for equipment?   Equipment.
6. Trout is the common name for many fresh water fish of what family?   Salmon.
7. What state in the USA has no fresh-water trout?   Florida.
8. Where would a fisherman look for a "Jitterbug" or "Hawaiian Wiggler"?   In a store that sells fishing equipment. They are lures.
9. Where did the pilot fish get its name?   Staying in close company with ships and larger fish.
10. Spawning trout will never bite.   True .... False (F).
11. Cape Cod was so named because of its many codfish. True (T)   False ....
12. The salmon, parr, and gulse are all the same fish. True (T)   False ....
13. The average casting distance for a nonprofessional is about 60'. True (T)   False ....

Fish Story

Question: The name of what lake means: "You fish on your side; we fish on our side, nobody fish in the middle?"

Answer: Lake Chargogagogmanchaugagogchwbunaguingamoug, located near Webster, Mass., three miles from the Connecticut line, on State Route 193. Transliterated from the Indian phrase, the fourteen syllable name is the longest identifying any place in the United States. The local population call it Lake Webster.

MISCELLANEOUS IDEAS: A "wanted" sign on the bulletin board

produced a sign painter for party posters, a pianist, guitarist, and accordion players.

Resident-assistants, when they have proved their ability and resourcefulness, are given improvised merit pins made in the craft shop. As a result of their help, it is possible to have more ward parties. In contests where teams won, one hospital found a special party to be the most popular prize — a table set with a table cloth and napkins, lighted candles where special sandwiches, cake, candy, and cocoa were served.

Other programs include musical request program of phonograph records or a band. Impromptu programs designated "anything goes" unearth an appreciable amount of talent and lead to a planned amateur show. A taffy-pull by the men, whose hands are stronger, receives an enthusiastic reception; pool tournaments and exhibition matches for the Home to watch are fun.

Chapter XV

QUIZZES

ORAL QUIZZES

Hɪɴᴛs ᴛᴏ ᴛʜᴇ Dɪsᴄᴜssɪᴏɴ Lᴇᴀᴅᴇʀ: Quizzes can serve in party plans or as questions starting discussion classes, using only those quizzes easy enough to keep it fun, not competitive.

Instead of the leader facing the group with the page of oral quizzes (which immediately puts up a barrier between the residents and the leader who has the answers), she gives the copy to the resident to read and has him direct the questions to the rest of the circle, discontinuing when the residents begin to tire of it.

Often it's necessary to give clues or help. One conundrum may suggest others which residents will contribute with rambling discussions developing.

Residents may take a page a day, and review the previous page discussed the day before.

Old Comic Strip Characters

This kid has grown from knee-pants days
To adolescent fun,
His face is brightly spotted
From playing in the sun.
Answer — Freckles and his Friends.

With muscles strong and x-ray eyes
Through steel or brick he goes.
You'll find him in the comic books
A hero each fan knows.
Answer — Superman.

'Mid wealth and riches he attempts
To lead a plain and simple life;
But corned beef, cabbage, and such things
Are frowned on by his wife.
Answer — Maggie and Jiggs.

He spurns his country sweetheart;
He's handsome and he's strong;
He's a simple bumpkin
Who always gets along.
Answer — Lil Abner.

A boasting, pompous, fat man this
With silk hat on his dome
With "h-rumph" and "egad" in his speech
He dominates his home.
Answer — Major Hoople.

His lock of hair just won't stay combed,
But he's really quite a man,
A sergeant with a wife and son.
The "Alley" thinks he's grand.
Answer — Gasoline Alley.

He's made the sandwich famous
And his dreams are quite delightful
The way he catches trains and busses
Is really very frightful.
Answer — Dagwood.

He never says a single word;
His antics are all funny;
He pantomimes most all folks' tricks;
He's really quite a honey.
Answer — Li'l Henry.

A gal with many fellows
And a suitor known as Mac,
She's really quite a steno,
And she went and joined the WAC.
Answer — Tillie the Toiler.

A champ of modest manner
He packs a mighty "right."
In the ring and in the Army
He's simple, but polite.
Answer — Joe Palooka.

With bulging muscles he abounds;
His food comes from a can;
He overpowers man and beast;
He's really quite a man.
Answer — Popeye.

Information Please

1. Is a hornet a wasp or a fly?   Wasp.
2. What is a philatelist?   Stamp collector.
3. What was Mark Twain's real name?   Samuel Clemens.
4. Name the Dionne quints.   Annette, Cecille, Emilie, Marie, and Yvonne.

5. How many squares has a checkerboard?   64.

6. What ingredient in food turns silver
black?   Sulphur.

7. How many children did Queen Vic-
toria have?   Nine.

8. On which coast of South America is
Peru?   West coast.

9. Which is on a US card, "Postal" or
"Post Card?"   Postal.

10. What typewriter keys are on either
side of W?   Q and E.

11. Do orchids grow from seeds?   Yes.

12. How many signed the Declaration of
Independence?   56.

13. What is the national flower of England?   Rose.

14. What state was the last one to join
the Union?   Hawaii.

15. What was President Wilson's first
name?   Thomas.

16. Give the common name of the plant,
"digitalis."   Foxglove.

17. What is the largest library in the
world?   Library of Congress.

18. Give another name for the growth,
"saguaro."   Giant cactus.

19. Who was Morpheus?   God of sleep.

Try These!

1. What is meant by the term "Southpaw"?
   A left-handed person.   A right-handed baseball player.

2. Which weighs more?
   A gallon of fresh water.   **A gallon of salt water.**

3. What is the Matterhorn?
   A mountain in the Alps.   The aged mother of a family.

4. Which one of the Great Lakes does not touch Canada?
   Michigan.   Erie.   Huron.

5. Which is larger?
   North America.   South America.

6. Is a tycoon:
   A small ape?   **A great business man?**   A tropical storm?

7. What dog is the result of crossing the mastiff and the greyhound?
   Great Dane.   Doberman pinscher.   Russian wolfhound.

8. If it takes three minutes to boil one egg, how long would it take to boil six?
   Three minutes.

9. How many players are on a football team?
   Nine.   **Eleven.**   Thirteen.

10. Is "syringa" the name of a:
    Drug?   **Flower?**   Surgical instrument?

11. Which produces the most wool?
    Canada.   **Australia.**   United States.

12. Which way around the earth is longer?
    Around the equator.   Around from pole to pole.

13. Where is Picardy?
    France.   England.   Ireland.

14. Which is the longest canal in the world?
    Panama.   **Suez.**   Canadian.

15. How many years is three score and ten?
    40   **70**   85

16. Is the Northern spy:
    A title of a Civil War story?   An apple?   A constellation?

17. Was the telephone invented by:
    Marconi?   Morse?   **Bell?**

18. What is the largest bird in the world?
    Albatross.   **Ostrich.**   Crane.

19. Is an earthquake tremor recorded on:
    A barograph?   A seismograph?   A tremolo?

20. Pygmies are natives of what continent?
    Australia.   Asia.   **Africa.**

Old Advertising Slogans

1. Keep that schoolgirl complexion.   **Palmolive.**
2. Chases dirt.   **Old Dutch.**
3. When it rains it pours.   **Morton's salt.**
4. Good to the last drop.   **Maxwell House Coffee.**
5. Hasn't scratched yet.   **Bon Ami.**
6. Eventually, why not now?   **Gold Metal Flour.**
7. From contented cows.   **Carnation milk.**
8. Digestible fat.   **Crisco.**
9. They satisfy.   **Chesterfield.**
10. Cover the earth.   **Sherwin William's paint.**
11. The flavor lasts.   **Wrigley chewing gum.**
12. No metal can touch you.   **Paris garters.**
13. Delicious and refreshing.   **Coca Cola.**
14. His master's voice.   **RCA Victor.**
15. Works while you sleep.   **Cascarets.**

16. The instrument of immortals.　　Steinway piano.
17. It floats.　　Ivory.
18. Ask the man who owns one.　　Packard.
19. A clean tooth never decays.　　Colgates.
20. There's a reason.　　Postum.
21. Time to retire.　　Fisk tires.
22. It's toasted.　　Lucky Strike.
23. For economical transportation.　　Greyhound.
24. The skin you love to touch.　　Woodbury.
25. The name that means everything in electricity.　　General Electric.

A Motor Romance

(Residents Guess the Word in Boldface)

Alice and her beau one day
Went riding in his **Chevrolet.**

Her beau was fat, his name was Frank,
And he was somewhat of a **crank.**

It was too bad he wasn't smarter
But he couldn't work the **starter.**

She showed him how, the little dear,
And also how to shift the **gear.**

Away they went, but something broke,
'Twas just a measley little **spoke.**

He fixed it with a piece of wire,
Then something popped — it was a **tire.**

'Twas mended soon, but next — ker — plop,
They struck a branch and smashed the **top.**

"Dear me," cried Alice, "That's too much!"
Then something happened to the **clutch.**

And next, poor Frank, unlucky dub,
Just grazed a rock and mashed a **hub.**

They crossed a brook and missed the ford,
And sank down to the **running board.**

"Oh, Frank," cried Alice with a squeal,
"I think we're going to lose a **wheel.**"

They climbed a hill, and then 'twas seen
The tank contained no **gasoline.**

They coasted downward toward the lake
But Frankie couldn't work the **brake.**

They struck a post a moment later
That almost wrecked the **radiator.**

So both climbed out and poor old Frank
Bought gasoline and filled the **tank.**

And gathered up from road and field
The fragments of the smashed **windshield.**

They fixed the engine tight and snug
And had to use a new **spark plug.**

Just then he slapped at a mosquito
And dropped a wrench on the **magneto.**

'Twas useless then to sweat and toil.
Nothing would run except the **oil.**

They journeyed home with Frankie pushin'
While Alice sobbed upon the **cushion.**

So poor Frank's hopes were doomed to blight
And Alice married **Willys-Knight.**

Let Me Think

1. What famous inventor was once a railroad newsboy?
   Henry Ford.   **Thomas A. Edison.** George Washington **Carver.**
2. What is a cowboy's piebald?
   His mottled horse.   His blanket.   His cooking **equipment.**
3. How many sides has an obelisk?
   Four.   Six.   Eight.
4. What is meant by propeller wash?
   Cleaning fluid.   Poor grade coffee. **Air current from a propeller.**
5. About what country is the famous book, **The Good Earth?**
   India.   **China.**   Japan.
6. How old are the juniper trees in Oregon estimated to be?
   500 years.   3000 years.   **8000 years.**
7. What food is boiled in lye?
   Hominy grits.   Pig's feet.   Some deep sea fish.
8. How large is an ordinary parachute?
   Eighteen feet.   **Twenty-four feet.** Thirty feet.
9. Where is the United States Military Academy?
   Annapolis.   Culver.   **West Point.**
10. What kind of type is Braille?
    Newspaper headline.   **For the blind.**   For small children.

11. If you are a gridiron fan, you like
    Waffles.   **Football.**   Fireside reading.
12. What portion of the earth's surface is covered with water?
    One-half.   **Three-fourths.**   Seven-eighths.
13. How long is the Panama Canal?
    Twelve miles.   Twenty-three and a half miles.   Fifty and four fourths miles.

Finish It

1. Experience is the **mother of learning.**
2. Familiarity breeds **contempt.**
3. All things come to him **who waits.**
4. A bird in the hand is **worth two in the bush.**
5. Music hath charms to **soothe the savage breast.**
6. Appearances are **deceitful.**
7. It takes two to make a **bargain or a quarrel.**
8. It is better to be safe **than sorry.**
9. Never grieve over **spilled milk.**
10. A watched pot **is long in boiling.**
11. Fine feathers **make fine birds.**
12. Possession is nine points **of the law.**
13. Wherever there is smoke **there's fire.**
14. Necessity is the **mother of invention.**
15. Speech is silver, **silence is golden.**
16. Never put off until tomorrow **what you can do today.**
17. Nothing ventured, **nothing gained.**
18. A stitch in time **saves nine.**
19. Honesty is the **best policy.**
20. A fool and his money **are soon parted.**
21. You can lead a horse to water **but you can't make him drink.**
22. Make hay while the **sun shines.**
23. Brevity is the **soul of wit.**
24. Manners make the **man.**
25. A rolling stone gathers **no moss.**
26. Still water **runs deep.**
27. Every rose has **its thorn.**

28. Easy come **easy go.**
29. Marry in haste and **repent at leisure.**
30. Paddle your **own canoe.**

Try Me

1. Who drove all the rats out of Hamelin Town? **Pied Piper.**
2. Is the accent on the first or second syllable in the word "adult"? **Second.**
3. Was Ty Cobb a famous baseball player or a humorous writer? **Baseball player.**
4. On what date is Armistice Day? **November 11.**
5. From what does gasoline come? **Petroleum.**
6. What is the one essential difference between a man's and a woman's suit jacket? **Buttoning.**
7. Which weighs more per bushel, wheat or apples? **Wheat.**
8. Where is the stratosphere? **Upper part of atmosphere.**
9. Which is farther north, Iceland or Lapland? **Lapland.**

Sports Quiz

1. What famous baseball player holds the home run record of sixty home runs in one season? **Babe Ruth.**
2. Of what great outfielder was it said that the only way to stop him on bases was to throw to third if he started for second? **Ty Cobb.**
3. Which of the following games originated in the United States — tennis, baseball, badminton, cricket? **Baseball.**
4. What famous evangelist was once a professional baseball player? **Billy Sunday.**
5. Jai Lai (Hy Ly) or Pelota is a game like checkers, chess, tennis, football, basketball, croquet, handball? **Handball and tennis.**
6. It originated in Ireland, Italy, South America, Cuba, India, Japan, Spain. **Spain.**
7. What famous football player was known as "The Galloping Ghost"? **Red Grange.**
8. If the player of the kicking side falls on the kickoff in the opposing team's end zone in a football game, does he

score a safety, a touchback, or a touchdown? **Touchdown.**

9. How many points does a football team score when it makes a safety? **Two.**

10. In the ordinary game of croquet are there seven, eight, or nine wickets? **Nine.**

11. Who are the two most famous archers in history and legend? **William Tell and Robin Hood.**

12. What champion heavyweight prizefighter was known as "Gentleman Jim"? **James Corbett.**

13. What are the positions in six-man football? **Center, two ends, quarterback, halfback, and fullback.**

14. Which is the older game, tennis or handball? **Handball.**

Penny Wise

You may be a winner. All the answers to these questions can be found on the penny. Take one out and look at it.

1. The name of a song **America.**
2. A privilege **Liberty.**
3. A small insect -B- **Bee.**
4. A part of Indian corn **Ear.**
5. Something denoting self **I.**
6. Part of a door **Lock of hair.**
7. A foreign fruit **Date.**
8. What ships sail on **C.**
9. A perfume **Scent.**
10. A Chinese beverage **T.**
11. A term of marriage **United.**
12. Part of a plant **Wheat leaves.**
13. A religious edifice **Temple on head.**
14. A messenger **One cent.**
15. A method of voting **No.**

Observation Quiz

1. How many times does the numeral one (1) or the word **one** appear on a one dollar bill — not counting the serial numbers? **Twenty-five.**

2. What suits of regular playing cards have one-eyed jacks? **Hearts and spades.**
3. Does the red or green light appear on top of a traffic signal? **Red.**
4. Whose face appears on a five-dollar bill? **Abe Lincoln.**
5. How many keys are there on a standard typewriter? **Forty-two.**
6. Do buttonholes of a man's shirt run vertically or horizontally? **Vertically.**
7. Is the hour hand above or below the minute hand on a watch? **Below.**
8. Do men's coats button to the right or the left? **Right.**
9. On which side is the bow on a man's hat? **Left.**
10. Whose face appears on a ten-dollar bill? **Alexander Hamilton.**
11. Which stripe appears at the top of the American flag, the red or the white? **Red.**
12. In a deck of playing cards, which king is in profile? **Diamonds.**
13. How are the pips of an eight arranged on playing cards?
14. On which side of the sink is the hot water usually found? **Left.**
15. Is the money-return slot of a public telephone on your right or left side? **Left.**
16. In which hand does the Statue of Liberty hold her torch? **Right.**
17. Does the eagle's head face right or left on a quarter? **Left.**
18. How many toes has a chicken? **Four.**

That's What I Was Going to Say!

1. What is an electrical transcription?

Phonographic record-ing for radio	An addition to a radio program.	Anything that fills in time on a program.

2. What was the gestapo?

Russian secret police.	**German secret police.**	Polish Underground.

3. About how long is the Lincoln Highway?

1,050 miles.	125 miles.	**3,140 miles.**

4. What is the national holiday of Canada?
   Dominion Day.   Labor Day.   July 4.

5. What mammal can live longest without water?
   Rat.   Camel.   Kangaroo.

6. Which is the most abundant metal?
   Aluminum.   Tin.   Zinc.

7. What is the oldest inhabited city in the world?
   Jerusalem.   Hong Kong.   **Damascus.**

8. What is a faux pas?
   A mistake.   Term of endearment.   Critical situation.

9. What was the first name of the Webster of dictionary fame?
   Daniel.   **Noah.**   John.

10. Who are the Untouchables?
    Highest born   **Outcasts in India.**   English residents
    East Indians   of India.

11. How much is 2½ times 2½?
    Five.   **Six and one fourth.**   Eight.

12. Which is the longest river in the United States?
    Missouri.   Mississippi.   Colorado.

13. What is the plural of moose?   **Moose.**

14. How many karats is pure gold?
    Eighteen.   **Twenty-four.**   Twenty-eight.

15. When was the presidential election in the United States first broadcast over the radio?
    1900.   **1920.**   1940.

16. Is a retina:
    A group of attendants?   **A part of the eye?**   A reproduction?

Do You Remember?

1. Who was the only man to knock out Jack Dempsey during his years as champion? **No one.**

2. Who did knock out John L. Sullivan? **Jim Corbett.**

3. Who was the only man to beat Willie Pep in competition? **Sandy Saddler.**

4. Who won the heavyweight boxing crown by a foul decision? **Jack Sharkey.**

5. Where is "a spot shot" used? **Pool.**

6. Where is a clay ball used by lobbing it against a backboard? **Jai lai.**

7. In what sport was there a "Louisville Slugger"? **Baseball.**

8. Who gave Joe Louis the worst beating in his entire career? **Max Schmelling.**

9. Who were the two great pitching brothers in the early '30's? **Dizzy and Paul Dean.**

10. Who was the "Beer Barrel"? **Tony Galento.**

11. Who was the greatest tennis champion of all time? **Big Bill Tilden.**

12. Who made top records in speed-boat racing and "sweet music"? **Guy Lombardo.**

13. Who was "Slinging Sammy"? **Sammy Baugh.**

14. Who refereed the greatest heavyweight matches from 1920-1940? **Arthur Donovan.**

15. Who established football as a great sport? **Walter Camp.**

16. Who played in more major league games than any man in baseball? **Lou Gehrig.**

17. Who was the greatest billiard man of all time? **Willie Hoppe.**

Food for Thought

What are appropriate foods for the following persons? Want an illustration? All right! What is an appropriate food for a taxi driver? **Cabbage.**

1. Jeweler? **Carrots.**

2. Prize fighter? **Duck.**

3. Plumber? **Leeks.**

4. Teacher? **Alphabet soup.**

5. Horticulturist? **Cauliflower.**

6. Policeman? **Beets.**

7. Traffic officer? **Jam.**

8. Actor? **Ham.**

9. Sailor? **Roe.**

10. Shoemaker? **Sole.**

11. Electrician? **Currants.**

12. Gambler? **Steaks.**

13. Newly weds? **Lettuce alone.**

14. Printer? **Pi (e).**

15. Wood cutter? **Chops.**

16. Real estate man? **Cottage cheese.**

17. Carpenter? **Hard tack.**
18. Fourth of July celebration? **Crackers.**
19. Chiropodist? **Corn.**
20. Baseball player? **Batter cake.**
21. Chess player? **Chess pie.**
22. The unemployed? **Meat loaf.**
23. Air conditioning engineer? **Chile.**
24. A marrying parson? **Pears.**
25. Stone mason? **Marble cake.**

Whose Tools Are These?

1. A micrometer is used by a	cook	**machinist**	baker
2. A colander is used by a	farmer	aviator	**cook**
3. An auger is used by a	**carpenter**	conductor	clergyman
4. A T-square is used by an	upholsterer	sculptor	**draftsman**
5. A conduit is used by an	**electrician**	druggist	barber
6. A cultivator is used by a	mason	**farmer**	fireman
7. A trowel is used by an	engineer	**mason**	fireman
8. A scalpel is used by a	printer	plumber	**surgeon**
9. Spigots are used by a	farmer	mailman	**plumber**
10. A spatula is used by a	druggist	**mason**	barber
11. A spindle is used by a	**weaver**	carpenter	dentist
12. A last is used by an	upholsterer	**cobbler**	dry cleaner
13. A ledger is used by a	sculptor	policeman	**accountant**
14. An easel is used by a	**painter**	blacksmith	interior decorator
15. A cant hook is used by a	grocer	**lumberjack**	painter

Guess What!

1. What animal lives the longest?
   Elephant.   **Tortoise.**   Hippopotamus.
2. What language is spoken in Switzerland?
   German.   **French.**   Italian.
3. When was the Nazi party formed?
   1918.   **1920.**   1932.
4. How many points is scored for a touchdown in football?
   Three.   **Six.**   Seven.

5. What is the national sport of Spain?
   Polo.   Horse racing.   **Bull fighting.**

6. What great city in U.S. is built on seven hills?
   San Francisco.   **Seattle.**   Memphis.

7. What is the name of the day celebrated by planting trees in a great many states?
   Arbor Day.   May Day.   Memorial Day.

8. In what one state are the highest and lowest points in the U.S.?
   Colorado.   Arizona.   **California.**

9. Is coral:
   Animal?   Vegetable?   Mineral?

10. What animal is rated next to man in intelligence?
    Horse.   Dog.   **Chimpanzee.**

11. What is a squab?
    A fat person.   Thickly stuffed cushion.   **Young pigeon.**

12. How many sides has a hexagon?
    Six.   Seven.   Eight.

13. What is the largest north-to-south stretch of land in the world?
    Asia.   Africa.   **The Americas.**

14. Which of the earth's oceans is the deepest?
    Pacific.   Atlantic.   Indian.

15. What percent of a watermelon is water?
    Thirty-five   Fifty-seven   **Ninety-two**
        per cent.   per cent.   **per cent.**

Hodgepodge Quiz

1. Is Phi Beta Kappa a social, professional, or **scholastic** fraternity?

2. The Ohio River forms the entire northern boundary of what state? **Kentucky.**

3. What colors are obtained by mixing (1) blue and yellow, (2) red and yellow, and (3) black and orange? **(1) Green. (2) Orange. (3) Brown.**

4. Why are pine trees less likely to be struck by lightning than any other trees? **The resin in the pine tree makes it a poor conductor.**

5. How many reindeer were there in the poem, **The Visit of St. Nicholas,** by Clement C. Moore? Can you name four of them? How does the poem begin? **Eight. Dasher, Dancer, Prancer, Vixen, Comet, Cupid, Donner and Blitzen. " 'Twas the night before Christmas and all through the house......"**

6. What character in nursery rhyme ate Christmas pie? **Little Jack Horner.**

7. What character in history was known as "The Father of His Country"? **George Washington.**

8. Which letters of the alphabet are used as Roman numerals? **I V X L D M C.**

9. Why is it that you see the lightning before you hear the thunder? **Because light travels faster than sound.**

Ask Me Another

1. The British Isles include what countries and islands? **Channel Island, England, Scotland, Northern Ireland, Wales, Isle of Man, etc.**

2. By what nickname was William Frederick Cody known? **Buffalo Bill.**

3. What is a fertile spot on a desert called? **Oasis.**

4. How many sheets of paper are there in a quire? **Twenty-four.**

5. Which has greater influence on the tide, the sun or the moon? **Moon.**

6. What does IQ stand for? **Intelligence Quotient.**

7. Which of the following are fresh-water fish: perch, shad, pike, salmon? **Perch, pike, salmon.**

8. Which weighs less, damp air or dry air? **Damp air.**

9. What and where is "Old Faithful"? **Geyser, Yellowstone National Park.**

Famous Similes

1. Deaf as a **post.**
2. Dumb as a **door bell.**
3. Bright as a **dollar.**

4. Smart as a **whip.**
5. Blind as a **bat.**
6. Brown as a **berry.**
7. Busy as a **bee.**
8. Clean as a **whistle.**
9. Clear as a **bell.**
10. Crazy as a **loon.**
11. Cross as a **bear.**
12. Dead as a **mackeral.**
13. Dry as a **bone.**
14. Fair as a **flower.**
15. Fat as a **pig.**
16. Fit as a **fiddle.**
17. Flat as a **pancake.**
18. Happy as a **lark.**
19. Hard as a **nail.**
20. Light as a **feather.**
21. Mad as a **hornet.**
22. Neat as a **pin.**
23. Nervous as a **cat's tail.**
24. Playful as a **kitten.**
25. Poor as **Job's turkey.**
26. Pretty as a **picture.**
27. Proud as a **peacock.**
28. Pure as a **lily.**
29. Quick as a **flash.**
30. Poor as a **churchmouse.**
31. Red as a **rose.**
32. Sharp as a **tack.**
33. Slippery as an **eel.**
34. Sly as a **fox.**
35. Sound as a **bell.**
36. Sour as a **lemon.**
37. Stiff as a **poker.**
38. Strong as an **ox or mule.**

39. Stubborn as a **mule**.
40. Thin as a **rail**.
41. Tight as a **drum**.

Front Page Mother Goose

Would you know some of the old Mother Goose rhymes if they were written in the style of a newspaper headline? For example, your morning or evening paper might use the following headline to explain how the marriage problem of Peter Pumpkin Eater was solved: "Pumpkin Shell Solves Marriage Question."

1. Mother Spanks Daughter for Sitting in Cinders. — **Polly Flinders.**
2. Boy Kisses Girls. Flees. — **Georgie Porgie.**
3. Man's Request for Taste of Pastry Denied. — **Simple Simon Met a Pieman.**
4. Farmer's Wife Attacked by Blind Rodents. — **Three Blind Mice.**
5. Boy Retires Wearing Trousers. — **Diddle Diddle Dumpling.**
6. Girl Frightened by Spider. — **Miss Muffet.**
7. Man and Horses Fail to Revive Crash Victim. — **Humpty Dumpty.**
8. Married Couple Hearty Eaters. — **Jack Sprat.**
9. Wool Supply Assured, Inquiry Reveals. — **Baa Baa Black Sheep.**
10. Unusual Pie Served Royalty. — **Four and Twenty Black Birds.**
11. Dogs Herald Beggar's Arrival. — **Hark Hark the Dogs Do Bark.**
12. Pig Thief Punished. — **Tom Tom the Piper's Son.**
13. Lady Mistreats Pony. — **I Had a Little Pony.**
14. Violinists Give Command Performance for King. — **Old King Cole**
15. Pupil Queried about Tardiness. — **Ten O'Clock Scholar.**
16. Woman Lacks Food. Dog Starves. — **Old Mother Hubbard.**
17. People's Taste for Porridge Vary. — **Pease Porridge Hot.**

18. Cripple Finds Bent Coin.

19. Queen's Tarts Stolen; Thief Repents after Beating.

20. Differences between Sexes Revealed.

21. Woman Visits Friends in Wheelbarrow.

22. Lamb Follows Mistress Everywhere.

23. Archer Confesses: Murder Solved.

24. Clock Strikes Hour, Frightens Rodent.

25. Cat Saved from Drowning by John Stout.

There Was a Crooked Man.

Queen of Hearts, She Made Some Tarts.

What Are Little Girls Made of?

Peter Peter Pumpkin Eater.

Mary Had a Little Lamb.

Who Killed Cock Robin?

Hickory Dickory Dock.

Ding Dong Bell, Pussy's in the Well.

Automobile Riddle

1. The fourteenth letter of the alphabet and the remains of a fire. **Nash.**
2. The name of a heavenly body. **Moon.**
3. Heavy twine. **Cord.**
4. A famous French explorer. **La Salle.**
5. A capital of one of the southern states. **Austin.**
6. The Spanish word for "river." **Rio.**
7. What early pioneers did when they came to a stream. **Ford.**
8. To be intoxicated and a trade. **Studebaker.**
9. Not a gentleman and five letters not in order that spell the name of a flower. **Cadillac.**
10. To duck when someone tries to strike you. **Dodge.**
11. A President who was assassinated. **Lincoln.**
12. A river in one of the Eastern states. **Hudson.**
13. A type of cracker. **Graham.**
14. A famous Indian chief. **Pontiac.**
15. One color of human hair. **Auburn.**
16. A famous violinist. **Chrysler.**

17. To penetrate and an Indian weapon. **Pierce Arrow.**

18. The Spanish explorer who discovered the Mississippi. **De Soto.**

19. A popular make of radio. **Crosley.**

20. A famous rock. **Plymouth.**

21. The first name of a President. **Franklin.**

22. Not young, a letter of the alphabet, a brand of oil. **Oldsmobile.**

23. A famous French statesman. **Lafayette.**

24. A term applied to a boxer weighing from 112 to 118 pounds. **Bantam.**

25. The Latin word for land and a carpenter's tool. **Terraplane.**

A Whiz of a Quiz

1. How much dirt is there in a hole eighteen inches square and one foot deep? **None.**

2. In what way are a girl's kisses like pickles in a bottle? **After you get the first one, the rest come easy!**

3. Why is the nose in the middle of the face? **Because it is the scenter.**

4. What is the difference between an elephant and a flea? **An elephant can have fleas, but a flea can't have elephants.**

5. What is the difference between opium and Abraham? **Opium is the juice of the poppy, and Abraham is the poppy of the Jews.**

6. Why is a dog biting his tail a good manager? **Because he makes both ends meet.**

7. What is the difference between an old penny and a new dime? **Nine cents.**

8. What are the little white things in a person's head that bite? **Teeth.**

9. What gets fat and never eats? **Balloon.** What's the biggest pencil in the world? **Pennsylvania.**

10. What is a sheep after it is six years old? **Seven years old.**

11. What is the most cowardly fruit? **A tomato. It hits you and runs!**

12. What is the longest sentence in the world? **"Go to prison for life."**

13. Who was the first man mentioned in the Bible? **Chap. I.**

14. What part of the day was Adam born? **He wasn't.**

15. What is full of holes but still holds water? **Sponge.**

16. What grows larger the more you take from it? **A hole.**

17. How can fishermen tell the weight of the fish they catch? **By the scales.**

18. Why does a policeman have brass buttons on his coat? **To button it!**

19. On what date is April first in Siam? **First of April.**

20. Who is the admiral of the Swiss navy? **They have no navy.**

21. Which is the other side of the street? **The side opposite the one on which you are.**

22. When the clock strikes thirteen, what time is it? **Time to have it repaired.**

23. What's always behind time? **The back of a clock.**

Who Am I???

1. As a young man I was known as the "Rail Splitter." **Lincoln.**

2. Because I flew alone, I was called the "Lone Eagle." **Lindbergh.**

3. P. T. Barnum named me the "Swedish Nightingale." **Jenny Lind.**

4. I am famed as the "Children's Poet." **Robert L. Stevenson.**

5. I wrote under the pen name of "Mark Twain." **Samuel Clemens.**

6. As a shepherd boy, I killed Goliath. **David.**

7. As the "Sage of Menlo Park," I lighted the world. **Edison.**

8. My soldiers called me "Old Hickory." **Andrew Jackson.**

9. As "Poor Richard" I was known for my almanac. **Benjamin Franklin.**

10. Believe it or not, I am known as "Believe it or not." **Ripley.**

11. As "Buffalo Bill," I fought many Indians. **William F. Cody.**

12. I was burned up as "The Maid of Orleans." **Joan of Arc.**

13. She told him, "Why don't you speak for yourself, John?" **Priscilla.**

14. I was a "Rough Rider" and a U.S. President. **Teddy Roosevelt.**

15. "I tank I go home; I vant to be alone." **Garbo.**

16. I am the world's most famous baby doctor. **Defoe.**

17. My record as the "King of Swat" is yet to be beaten. **Babe Ruth.**

18. I formulated the theory of relativity. **Einstein.**

19. My nickname is "The Little Corporal." **Napoleon.**

20. I go to Africa and "bring them back alive." **Frank Buck.**

21. As the "Brown Bomber" I am known for my "Dead Pan." **Joe Louis.**

22. I made the world's most famous night ride. **Paul Revere.**

23. As a football player, I wore the number "77." Tom Harmon; **Red Grange.**

24. I composed **"Alexander's Ragtime Band." Berlin.**

25. I as known as the "Greatest Showman on Earth." **P. T. Barnum.**

26. As the "Little Giant," I debated with Lincoln. **Douglas.**

27. I shot an apple off my son's head with an arrow. **William Tell.**

28. I am Daffy's brother but not as dizzy as you think. **Dizzy Dean.**

29. I was known as "The Father of His Country." **Washington.**

30. I said, "Give me liberty, or give me death." **Patrick Henry.**

31. I am a poet, but they named a cigar after me. **Robert Burns.**

32. I was called "Silent Cal." **Calvin Coolidge.**

33. I am an Indian princess who saved a man named Smith. **Pocahontas.**

34. Because of my big nose, I am called "Schnozzola." **Jimmy Durante.**

Oldsters' Musical Quiz

1. What did I hold "on my knee" when "I went to Alabama" to see Susanna? **Banjo.**
2. "You may search everywhere but none can compare," with what? **"My Wild Irish Rose."**
3. What color was "the bonnet with the blue ribbons on it?" **Grey.**
4. What time of the year am I "coming back to you" in the Rockies? **Springtime.**
5. What's breaking up that "old gang of mine?" **Wedding bells.**
6. With whom did Casey waltz? **Strawberry blonde.**
7. Where would you like to be lost? **In each other's arms.**
8. "In the evening by the moonlight" what did you hear singing? **Darkies.**
9. Where do the buffaloes roam? **On the range.**
10. "Down in lovers' lane we'll wander, sweetheart, you and I." Name this song. **"Wait 'til the Sun Shines, Nellie."**
11. "Coming for to carry me home," a band of what is coming after me? **Angels.**
12. For whom did you buy "a home and ring and everything?" **Margie.**
13. What did he drink "in a tavern in the town?" **Wine.**
14. Name the title of the song which goes "Come and sit by my side if you love me, Do not hasten to bid me adieu. . . ." **"Red River Valley."**
15. For how many was the bicycle built? **Two.**
16. How did the man on the flying trapeze float through the air? **With the greatest of ease.**
17. What did Dinah blow? **Horn.**
18. Who was in the kitchen with Dinah? **Someone.**
19. Where did I first meet you? **"Down by the Old Mill Stream."**
20. Who was told to lay that pistol down? **Pistol Packin' Mama.**
21. What were you doing in the cabaret when Pistol Packin' Mama came in? **Drinkin' beer.**

So You Think You're Clever

1. If three cats can kill three rats in three minutes, how long will it take 100 cats to kill 100 rats? **Three minutes.**

2. I have two current US coins in my hand. Together they total 55¢. One is not a nickel. What are the coins? **Fifty cent piece and a nickel.**

3. A little Indian and a big Indian are walking down a path. The little Indian is the big Indian's son. The big Indian is not the little Indian's father. Who is it? **Mother.**

4. Which is correct: 8 and 8 is 15, or 8 and 8 are 15? **Neither.**

5. Is it legal for a man to marry his widow's sister? **No.**

6. There are ten black stockings and ten white stockings in a drawer. If you reach into the drawer in the dark, what is the minimum number of stockings you must take out before you are sure of having a pair that match? **Three.**

7. I have two minutes in which to catch a train and two miles to go. If I go the first mile at the rate of thirty miles per hour, at what rate must I go the second mile in order to catch the train? **Missed train.**

8. The number of eggs in a basket doubles every minute. The basket is full of eggs in an hour. When was it half full? **Fifty-nine minutes.**

9. A shepherd had seventeen sheep. All but nine died. How many did he have left? **Nine.**

10. Two fathers and two sons each shot a duck and none of them shot the same duck. Only three ducks were shot, why? **Grandfather, father, and son.**

11. What is the smallest number of ducks that could swim in this formation? Two ducks in front of a duck, two ducks behind a duck, and a duck between two ducks? **Three.**

12. Which would you prefer, a truck load of nickels or a half truck load of dimes? **Dimes.**

13. We all know that there are twelve — 1¢ stamps in a dozen, but how many 2¢ stamps are there in a dozen? **Twelve.**

14. A rope ladder ten feet long is hanging over the side of a ship. The rungs are a foot apart, and the bottom rung is resting on the surface of the water. The tide rises at the rate of six inches an hour. When will the first three rungs be covered with water? **Never.**

15. "A" owns a peacock. If the peacock laid an egg in "B's" yard, who would own the egg, "A" or "B"? **Peacocks don't lay eggs.**

Supermarket

(Found in stores)

Leader: Give the first letter and the number of letters.
Residents: Fill in the blanks.

1.	A chart	**M a p**
2.	Something to catch mice	**T r a p**
3.	To dine	**S u p**
4.	Flesh foods	**M e a t s**
5.	Hard fat	**S u e t**
6.	A band or fastening	**S t r a p**
7.	A coarse file	**R a s p**
8.	A Scottish cap	**T a m**
9.	An afternoon beverage	**T e a**
10.	A covering for the face	**M a s k**
11.	A pocketbook	**P u r s e**
12.	Bartletts	**P e a r s**
13.	A canned meat (trade name)	**S p a m®**
14.	A garden tool	**R a k e**
15.	A hair pad	**R a t**
16.	An ice runner	**S k a t e**
17.	A flat cushion	**M a t**
18.	A porterhouse	**S t e a k**
19.	A tone softener	**M u t e**
20.	A musical instrument	**U k e**
21.	A household animal	**P e t**

What to Wear

What is appropriate material for the following people to wear?

1. The artist?   Canvas.
2. The dairyman?   Cheesecloth.
3. The editor?   Prints.

4. The banker? Checks.
5. The gardener? Lawn.
6. The Scotchman? Plaid.
7. The hunter? Duck.
8. The barber? Haircloth.
9. The fisherman? Net.
10. The government official? Red tape.
11. The prisoner? Stripes.
12. The minister? Broadcloth.
13. The bald man? Mohair.
14. The jeweler? Goldcloth.
15. The undertaker? Crepe.
16. The filling station employee? Oilcloth.
17. The inventor? Patent leather.

Fishing

Here are some well known fish. How many can you identify or catch? Here are the clues:

1. A struggling fish. **Flounder.**
2. A fraudulent or cheating fish. **Shark.**
3. A fish of precious metal. **Gold.**
4. Man's best friend. **Dog.**
5. A royal fish. **King.**
6. A heavenly fish. **Angel.**
7. A fish in the band. **Drum.**
8. Animal almost extinct that roamed the plains. **Buffalo.**
9. A household pet. **Cat.**
10. A fish in a bird cage. **Perch.**
11. A member of the barbershop quartet. **Bass.**
12. Some boats have them. **Sail.**
13. Used by a fencer. **Sword.**
14. Seen at night. **Star.**
15. Good with bread and butter. **Jelly.**
16. An evil fish. **Devil.**

17. Colorless fish. **White.**

18. A popular alphabet code for stores that deliver. **Cod.**

19. A process for refining metal. **Smelt.**

20. Warms the earth. **Sun.**

Games for Sportsmen

Are you a good sportsman? Below are fifty questions about sports, pastimes, and indoor games.

A. Name the game in which the following expressions are used:

1. Fore   (Golf)
2. Slide   (Baseball)
3. Break   (Boxing)
4. Service   (Tennis)
5. Sweep   (Hockey)
6. Checkmate   (Chess)
7. Double   (Baseball)
8. Tallyho   (Fox Hunting)
9. Fifteen two   (Cribbage)
10. First down   (Football)

B. Name the game which is started in each of the following ways:

1. Jump at center   (Basketball)
2. Kick off   (Football)
3. Play for serve   (Tennis)
4. Low cut deals   (Cribbage)
5. Break the balls   (Pool)
6. Face off   (LaCrosse)
7. Tee off   (Golf)
8. Bell rings   (Boxing)
9. On the mark   (Racing)
10. Batter up   (Baseball)

C. Name the sport in which each of the following is forbidden or illegal:

1. Shiny buttons on uniform   (Fencing)
2. Leg before   (Track)
3. Reneging   (Cards)
4. Hooking   (Hockey)
5. Improving lie   (Golf)
6. Moving into check   (Chess)
7. Feet past limit   (Bowling)
8. Touching net   (Tennis)
9. Touching ball with arm   (Volleyball)
10. Moistening ball   (Baseball)

D. Name the sport in which each of the following is used:

1. Epee   (Fencing)
2. Brassie   (Golf)
3. Bird   (Badminton)
4. Silks   (Racing)
5. Rosin bag   (Baseball)
6. Eight ball   (Pool)
7. Fly   (Fishing)
8. Touching net   (Basketball)
9. Touching ball with arm   (Soccer football)
10. Moistening ball   (Water polo)

E. Name the game which is measured off by each of the following:

1. Rounds   (Boxing)
2. Rubber   (Cards)
3. Innings   (Baseball)
4. Frames   (Bowling)
5. Periods   (Basketball)
6. Sets   (Tennis)
7. 18 holes   (Golf)
8. 120 holes   (Cribbage)
9. Quarters   (Football)

WRITTEN QUIZZES

It isn't usually possible in the Homes to have written quizzes mimeographed; however, in the following quizzes, the quiz or part of the quiz can be written on a large blackboard facing the group of residents and can be done orally.

Another use of written quizzes can be made with big sheets of butcher's paper taped on a wall and the quiz printed or written in large letters in crayon for residents as a group to solve together.

Other Homes use parts of a quiz in the Home newspaper or on a bulletin board in a contest to be done individually.

Rexographed or mimeographed quizzes which are distributed, slow down a group activity when residents are asked to settle down with paper and pencil. Sheets may be distributed and collected at some later date if the residents like the idea of individual competition.

Cached Food

There are twenty-one different fruits and vegetables hidden in the following telegram. How many of them can you find? They may be located in one word or connecting word. They are in their proper sequence. Disregard punctuation marks.

S.E. 308 D.L. PD-TDS   SANTA MONICA, CALIF. 16
TO: MRS. O.K. RAVEN
     1061 FIFTH AVE.
     NEW YORK, N.Y.   DATE: JULY 12, 1963

HAVE RUN INTO LIVE REAL-ESTATE AGENT AND BOUGHT HOUSE ON BEACH. BECAUSE OF HEAVY SCHEDULE I CAN'T RETURN. I PRESUME YOU WILL BE AN ANGEL AND CLOSE THE NEW YORK HOUSE ALONE. FIND LIVING HERE VERY CHEAP. PLEASE CALL PLUMBER AND HAVE HIM TURN OFF WATER AND LOOK INTO RANGE IN KITCHEN. ALSO HAVE PHONE COMPANY DISCONTINUE OUR NUMBER. RYE AND SCOTCH PLENTIFUL. IT'S A SUBLIME SPOT. A TORN PAIR OF PANTS FOR ME. FOR YOU A BATHING SUIT AND CAPE. ACHIEVES THE END I'VE ALWAYS LONGED FOR. AM IN FINE

CONDITION. I ONLY HOPE YOU AND THE KIDS ARE THE SAME. WHEN I THINK OF THE PLAY AND MY OWN PART, I CHOKE WITH TEARS. BUT IN THE THEATRE MY HEAD BEGINS TO SPIN. ACHES AND PAINS CONSTANTLY RECUR. RANTING SHAKESPEARE AND TEMPESTUOUS BEETHOVEN ARE NOT FOR ME. I WILL SPEAK TO YOU ON SATURDAY AND WILL SEND YOU SNAPS OF THE NEW HOUSE AND THE MAGNIFICENT BEACH.

ARDENTLY YOURS
OLLY

1. OKRA ....
2. DATE ....
3. OLIVE ....
4. TURNIP ....
5. BEAN ....
6. APPLE ....
7. PLUM ....
8. ORANGE ....
9. BERRY ....
10. LIME ....

11. POTATO ....
12. PEACH ....
13. ENDIVE ....
14. ONION ....
15. ARTICHOKE ....
16. SPINACH ....
17. CURRANT ....
18. PEAR ....
19. BEET ....
20. PEA ....

Mathematics — Front and Center

Can you fill in the blanks with numbers one through nine so that you will get fifteen whether you add horizontally, vertically, or diagonally?

	3	8	= 15
9		1	= 15
2	7		= 15

= 15 = 15 = 15

Okay! Now try this one with twenty-five squares. This adds up to sixty-five.

11	18	25		9
10		19	21	3
4	6	13	20	
23	5		14	16
	24	1	8	15

Now for a really hard one. This adds up to 121.

22		40	49	2	11	20
	23	32	41	43	3	12
13	15		33	42	44	1
5	14	16	25		36	45
46	6	8		26	35	37
38	47	7	9	18		29
30	39	48	1	10	19	

Make up some others for the rest of us.

Automobiles

These are the cars hidden in these squares. Letter may be

O	R	E	T	R	O	D	E	W	X
V	L	H	C	L	S	L	L	I	A
R	E	D	E	Y	L	R	Y	S	M
L	A	T	S	D	P	O	C	E	D
D	N	U	O	M	U	D	R	G	R
A	T	N	D	O	A	H	A	E	O
S	Z	C	E	B	U	R	K	N	F
Y	H	R	U	A	I	N	C	L	I
R	C	E	A	C	K	L	A	F	A
U	R	M	D	I	L	E	R	P	T

Fig. 38

used more than once but not in the same word. Letters must be touching in sequence — for a start: OLDSMOBILE is marked in the upper left. You may be taken for a ride, because some of them are very old.

1. Oldsmobile	12. Dodge
2. Willys	13. Franklin
3. Ford	14. Packard
4. Fiat	15. Crosley
5. Cadillac	16. Hudson
6. Buick	17. Mercury
7. Maxwell	18. Star
8. Reo	19. Stutz
9. Mack	20. Nash
10. Overland	21. Hupmobile
11. Studebaker	

The Proverbial Quiz

Scrambled Proverbs

Parts of two proverbs are combined into one in the following ten scrambled proverbs. List the twenty correct proverbs.

1. A stitch in time / is worth two in the bush.
2. Practice / makes the heart grow fonder.
3. Misery loves / a fool and his money.
4. All things come to him who / catches the worm.
5. Birds of a feather / spoil the broth.
6. Actions speak louder / when the cat's away.
7. You can't have your cake and / lie on it.
8. A rolling stone / is as good as a mile.
9. Fools rush in / before they are hatched.
10. Still water / has a silver lining.

1. A stitch in time saves nine.
2. A bird in the hand is worth two in the bush.
3. Practice makes perfect.
4. Absence makes the heart grow fonder.
5. Misery loves company.
6. A fool and his money are soon parted.
7. All things come to him who waits.
8. The early bird catches the worm.
9. Birds of a feather flock together.
10. Too many cooks spoil the broth.
11. Actions speak louder than words.
12. When the cat's away the mice will play.
13. You can't have your cake and eat it too.
14. You've made your bed, now lie in it.
15. A rolling stone gathers no moss.
16. A miss is as good as a mile.
17. Fools rush in where angels fear to tread.
18. Don't count your chickens before they are hatched.
19. Still water never runs deep.
20. Every cloud has a silver lining.

Crime — without Punishment

Each person listed in the column at the right is mentioned in the column at the left. Your job is to match them up correctly.

Put correct letter from column at right in parenthesis at left margin. (The author has filled them in correctly.)

(e) 1. He was known as "Pretty Boy."

    a.   Robin Hood

(d) 2. He wrote **Crime and Punishment.**

    b.   Al Capone

(c) 3. Public Enemy Number One was killed in an alley near a Chicago theatre.

    c.   John Dillinger

(j)	4.	He killed all his wives.	d.	Feodor Dostoievsky
(f)	5.	He was a dapper, love-able safecracker in O. Henry fiction.	e.	Floyd
(b)	6.	Once king pin of the underworld, he was sent to Alcatraz for income tax evasion.	f.	Jimmy Valentine
(g)	7.	He created a famous monster.	g.	Frankenstein
(i)	8.	He kidnaped Lindbergh's baby.	h.	Cain
(l)	9.	In a famous French novel he stole a loaf of bread.	i.	Bruno Hauptmann
(n)	10.	He boasted that he was the world's greatest imposter.	j.	Blue Beard
(h)	11.	We know him as the first murderer.	k.	Tom, the Piper's Son
(m)	12.	They stole two white women.	l.	Jean Valjean
(o)	13.	He haunted an opera house.	m.	Apache Indians
(a)	14.	He was a famous English outlaw who robbed the rich, gave to the poor.	n.	Prince Michael Romanoff
(k)	15.	He stole a pig "and away he run."	o.	Phantom of the Opera

Match 'em up Quiz
(None are used twice)

1. Ably	21. Life	4-40	Bookworm
2. Ball	22. Like	6-9	Crawfish
3. Bill	23. Ling	7-34	Doorstep
4. Book	24. Lock	8-5	Downcast
5. Cast	25. Long	10-2	Football
6. Craw	26. Maid	11-24	Forelock
7. Door	27. Main	12-3	Handbill
8. Down	28. Mast	13-32	Hardship

9. Fish	29. Milk	15-18	Headland
10. Foot	30. Need	17-36	Homeward
11. Fore	31. Over	19-1	Laudably
12. Hand	32. Ship	21-22	Lifelike
13. Hard	33. Side	27-28	Main mast
14. Haul	34. Step	29-26	Milkmaid
15. Head	35. Suck	30-20	Needless
16. Hold	36. Ward	31-14	Overhaul
17. Home	37. With	33-25	Sidelong
18. Land	38. Wood	35-23	Suckling
19. Laud	39. Work	37-16	Withhold
20. Less	40. Worm	38-39	Woodwork

Famous Numbers

Fill in the correct number.

1. His better **half.**
2. The Unholy **Three.**
3. At the stroke of **twelve.**
4. **Seven** year itch.
5. **Thousand** island dressing.
6. House of **Seven** Gables.
7. Pieces of **eights.**
8. **Twentieth** Century Limited.
9. The **Three** Musketeers.
10. **Four** Wheel Drive.
11. The Gay **Nineties.**
12. The **fourth** dimension.
13. "**Thirty-two Forty** or fight."
14. **Seven** Keys to Baldpate.
15. A **four** flusher.
16. The **three** R's.
17. Tale of **Two** Cities.
18. Fair, Fat and **forty.**
19. **Seven** come **eleven.**
20. **Seventh** inning stretch.
21. He sailed the **seven** seas.
22. The **thirteen** colonies.
23. Tea for **two.**
24. **Ten**nessee.
25. **Three** wise men.
26. **Seventh** Day Adventist.
27. **Twelfth** Night.
28. Cat of **nine** tails.
29. Useless as a **fifth** wheel.
30. **Ten** nights in a barroom.
31. **Seven** men on a dead man's chest.
32. **Two** is company, **three's** a crowd.
33. **Seven** wonders of the world.
34. **Three** blind mice.
35. Ali Baba and the **forty** thieves.
36. The baker's dozen, **thirteen.**
37. **Four**-in-hand.
38. **Three** cheers.
39. Friday the **thirteenth.**
40. A **100** per cent American.
41. The roaring **twenties.**
42. "A" number **one.**
43. Around the World in **Eighty** Days.
44. "You were **sixteen,** my village queen."
45. **Seven** years of bad luck.
46. The **eleventh** hour, over the top.
47. Sweet **sixteen** and never been kissed.
48. "Into the valley of death rode the **400.**"
49. **Four** and **twenty** blackbirds.
50. The **three** bears.
51. Drawn and **quartered.**
52. The Armistice, **eleventh** hour, **eleventh** month, and **eleventh** day.
53. "The night has a **thousand** eyes, the day but **one.**"
54. New York's **Fifth** Avenue shops.
55. **One, two,** buckle my shoe.
56. A cat has **nine** lives.
57. The first **100** years are the hardest.
58. Rain before **seven,** dry before **eleven.**
59. It rained **forty** days and **forty** nights.

Word Ladder

Change **one** letter of the word in column "B" to get the succeeding word; **no skipping** because each word is built on the one immediately preceding it. Here goes — watch the definitions!

A	B
1. Throw forcibly	Fling
2. Bandage for broken limb	Sling — Now you are on your own!
3. Undignified words	(Slang)
4. Incline — at an angle	(Slant)
5. To establish - or to sow	(Plant)
6. To smooth wood with a tool	(Plane)
7. A flat or shallow table dish	(Plate)
8. A kind of rock	(Slate)
9. To speak or make an assertion	(State)
10. A fixed gaze	(Stare)
11. To enjoy in common with others	(Share)
12. Land on edge of the sea	(Shore)
13. Small routine job	(Chore)
14. Selected	(Chose)
15. Pursue	(Chase)
16. To stop — or discontinue	(Cease)
17. To rent	(Lease)
18. Smallest degree	(Least)
19. Animal	(Beast)
20. Loud, sudden noise	(Blast)

A Puzzling if-so Test

1. If blackberries are green when they are ripe, write H at the right hand side of this test. If not, write X. **H**

2. If black cows give white milk that makes yellow butter, write A at the right hand side. If not, write Y. **A**

3. If a regulation football field is just 90 yards long from goal to goal, write Z to the right. if not, write V. **V**

4. If paper is made out of wood, write E to the right. If not, write a zero.   **E**

5. If an airplane can travel faster than an automobile, write A. If not, write the number four.   **A**

6. If summer is warmer than winter, write G in the margin. If not, write R.   **G**

7. If Longfellow wrote "Twinkle, Twinkle, Little Star," write S in the margin. If not, write O.   **O**

8. If candy is sweeter than lemons, write O in the margin. If not, write the number three.   **O**

9. If Beethoven wrote "**Moonlight Sonata**," write D in the margin. If not, write the number four.   **D**

10. If the climate in Siberia is warmer than it is in Florida, write X in the margin. If not, write T.   **T**

11. If the printing press was first invented by an American, write Z in the margin. If not, write I.   **I**

12. If New York City is the capital of New York State, write A in the margin. If not, write M.   **M**

13. If baseball is a major sport, write E in the margin. If not, write O.   **E**

The name of all fifty states can be found among these letters. The name of the state is sometimes read forward, at other times backward, up, down, or diagonally. Circle the state when you locate it.

S	T	T	E	S	U	H	C	A	S	S	A	M	T	R	S	M	Z	A	O	R	U
R	E	T	S	K	C	I	K	P	L	B	V	R	S	Y	A	V	E	M	A	A	W
A	N	O	Z	I	R	A	I	N	I	G	R	I	V	T	S	E	W	I	D	N	Y
A	I	N	R	O	F	I	L	A	C	U	A	Z	X	Y	S	R	G	N	I	A	K
N	O	T	G	N	I	H	S	A	W	L	N	A	B	S	T	M	E	N	R	I	C
S	O	U	T	H	D	A	K	O	T	A	N	E	E	J	J	O	O	E	O	S	U
M	A	R	Y	L	A	N	D	L	M	I	H	N	W	N	O	N	R	S	L	I	T
O	P	U	T	A	H	R	S	T	L	N	N	U	E	J	V	T	G	O	F	U	N
A	K	A	X	H	O	A	W	O	I	E	Y	Z	A	V	E	R	I	T	S	O	E
K	R	L	S	B	C	D	R	E	T	F	C	I	J	K	A	R	A	A	X	L	K
S	O	A	A	I	N	A	V	L	Y	S	N	N	E	P	M	D	S	N	O	P	E
A	Y	S	X	H	C	S	R	N	A	G	I	H	C	I	M	N	A	E	T	U	R
R	W	K	E	H	O	W	Y	O	M	I	N	G	V	S	A	X	Y	S	Y	A	H
B	E	A	T	C	E	M	F	I	L	G	H	T	I	K	L	I	K	I	E	O	O
E	N	U	K	L	M	N	A	H	M	I	H	E	R	C	A	R	T	N	H	D	D
N	O	R	T	H	D	A	K	O	T	A	N	A	G	L	B	N	I	D	U	A	E
S	R	I	R	U	O	S	S	I	M	I	T	A	I	S	A	A	S	I	N	R	I
N	E	W	H	A	M	P	S	H	I	R	E	B	N	O	M	O	R	A	E	O	S
S	G	I	P	P	I	S	S	I	S	S	I	M	I	V	A	V	W	N	S	L	L
Y	O	C	I	X	E	M	W	E	N	D	E	L	A	W	A	R	E	A	X	O	A
X	N	I	S	N	O	C	S	I	W	R	T	S	A	N	A	T	N	O	M	C	N
T	T	U	C	I	T	C	E	N	N	O	C	S	I	O	N	I	L	L	I	X	D

INFORMATION ON RESOURCES
AND MATERIALS[1]

There are many worthwhile and informative booklets which can be obtained from both the federal and state governments. Catalogues can be secured in most cases.

Government Printing Office
Washington, D. C.

U.S. Dept. of Health, Education and Welfare
Washington, D. C.

Library of Congress
Washington, D. C.

The State Chamber of Commerce in a state capitol building usually has informative booklets. The United Nations and foreign embassies can supply information and materials about their respective countries, often free of charge.

Film Sources

"Guide to Visual Aids for Physical Education, Sports and Recreation"

The Athletic Institute
209 South State Street
Chicago 4, Illinois

"Selected Motion Pictures"
Associated Films, Inc.
347 Madison Avenue
New York 17, New York

Film Catalogue
Audio-Visual Aids
Library
Penn State University
University Park, Pennsylvania

---

[1]Credit for the following list is given to the Office for the Aging, Pennsylvania, Dept. of Public Welfare, Harrisburg, Pennsylvania.

Film Catalogue
Metropolitan Life Insurance Company
1 Madison Avenue
New York 10, New York

"Educators Guide to Free Films"
Educators Progress Service
Randolph, Wisconsin

Film Catalogue on Free Films
The Sterling Movies, Inc.
6 East 39th Street
New York, New York

For Residents with Some Use of Their Hands

For craft materials, solicit materials from local or national manufacturers. A prepared letter might tell just how one would use what they might send in recreation and rehabilitation programs.

Department stores or display departments might contribute materials left over from window displays.

Don't miss opportunities to visit the following:
Home furnishing shows
Garden shows (ask for donations of pots and plants)
Funeral parlors for flowers and pots
Auto shows (for small model cars)
Decorators' shows (for samples)
Plastic shows (for samples)
Architectural shows (make your request and how you plan to use the materials)

Leather

General Leather Craft (manual)
McKnight and McKnight
Bloomington, Illinois

Doodle Page. Free catalogue available
Art Handicraft Company
26 Frankfort Street
New York, New York

Catalogue
Osborn Brothers Supply Co.
223 West Jackson Blvd.
Chicago, Illinois

Catalogue
> J. C. Larson Company
> 280 South Tripp Avenue
> Chicago 24, Illinois

Catalogue
> Dearborn Leather Company
> 8625 Linwood
> Detroit 6, Michigan

Catalogue
> Tandy Leather Company
> P. O. Box 791
> Fort Worth, Texas

Catalogue
> Rosenblum Leather Company
> 2116 N. 15th Street
> Sheboygan, Wisconsin

Catalogue
> Arts and Crafts Dist., Inc.
> 9520 Baltimore Avenue
> College Park, Maryland

Crocheting, Knitting and Tatting

Catalogue, **Cutting, Sewing and Handicraft**
> Lee Wards Company
> Elgin, Illinois

Catalogue
> Nelson Knitting Company
> Rockford, Illinois

> Larkin Enterprises
> Box 424
> Scottsbluff, Nebraska
> "Petite Doll Knitting Book" 40¢

> Kessenick Looms and Knit Shop, Inc.
> 7463 Harwood Avenue
> Wauwatosa 13, Wisconsin
> Yarn of all kinds

> Lilly Mills Company
> Shelby, North Carolina

> Putnam Dye Company
> Quincy, Illinois

Plastics

Catalogues available from:
D. W. Cone Plastic Company
7401 Marillac Drive
St. Louis 21, Mo.

Cope Plastics Inc.
Highway 11
Godfrey, Illinois 62035

Plastic Parts and Sales
1157 S. Kings Highway
St. Louis, Mo.

Ceramics

American Art Clay Company
4717 West 16th Street
Independence Square

Basketry

Weaving the New Basket

Ladies Home Journal
Curtis Publishing Co.
Independence Square
Philadelphia 5, Penn.

Stenciling

Do It Yourself Catalogue available

The American Crayon Co.
1706 Hayes Avenue
Sandusky, Ohio

Textiles and Weaving

New Key to Weaving $12.00 a copy

Bruce Publishing Company 1966
400 N. Broadway
Milwaukee, Wisconsin 53201

Weaving Crafts

McKnight and McKnight Company
Bloomington, Illinois

Catalogues Available:
J. L. Hammet Company
Syracuse, New York

Brodfead and Garrett Company
4570 East 71st Street
Cleveland, Ohio

Howard Bradshaw and Company
Box 1103
Spartanburg, S. Carolina

Reed and Raffia

American Reedcraft Corp.
417 Lafayette Avenue
Box 154
Hawthorne, N. J. 07507
Cane circular which is free

Supply Firms' Addresses

Wilson Arts and Crafts
323 South West 4th Street
Faribault, Minnesota
Silk screen, finger painting and textiles

Handcrafters
Waupun, Wisconsin
Craft supplies

Cleveland Crafts of New York
4 East 16th Street
New York 3, New York
Craft supplies

J. L. Hammet Company
290 Main Street
Cambridge, Mass. 02142
Handicraft supplies, art materials, awards

Beckley-Cardy Company
1900 North Narragansett
Chicago, Illinois 60639

The Castolite Company
Woodstock, Illinois
Laminating material
Liquid plastics and fiberglass.

Louell Products Company
246 Fifth Avenue
New York, New York
Laminating material and kits.

Mosaic Crafts
80 West 3rd Street (off Wash. Square)
New York, New York
Everything in mosaics and instruction.

Walco Bead Company
37 West 37th Street
New York, New York
All kinds of beads.

Binney and Smith
380 Madison Avenue
New York, New York
All kinds of art supplies.

B. F. Drakenfeld & Co., Inc.
45 Park Place
New York, New York
Kilns -ceramic supplies.

Stewart Clay Company
133 Mulberry Street
New York City
Ceramic equipment ,
glass colors and clays.

Jack Wolfe & Company
62 Horatio Street
New York City
Ceramic supplies — clays.

O. P. Craft Company
Sandusky, Ohio
Wooden boxes and craft items for decorating etc.

S and S Leather Company
Colchester, Connecticut
Crafts, reeds, mosaics, chenille.

American Crayon Company
Education Department
9 Rockefeller Plaza
New York, New York
Crayola crafts.

Dennison Manufacturing Company
300 Howard Street
Framingham, Massachusetts
Paper crafts and decorations,
leaflets sent on request

American Handicrafts Company
20 West 14th Street
New York, N.Y. 10011
Arts and crafts supplies

Delco Craft Center Inc.
30081 Stephenson Highway
Madison Heights, Michigan 48071

Economy Crafts
47-11 Francis Lewis Blvd.
Flushing, New York

Carpentry

Workbench
P.O. Box 5965
Kansas City, Mo.

A magazine which includes patterns for carpentry; patio chair, projector stand, bookshelf, contemporary coffee table, straddle cabinet, curve back chair, patio bench, mousetrap mail box, telephone stool and recreation table, etc.; five issues for $1.00.

Easi-Bild Pattern Company, Inc.
Pleasantville, New York
Patterns for large furniture items

Craftsman's Wood Service Company
2727 South Mary Street
Chicago 8, Illinois
Veneer wood; send 25¢ for catalogue

Giles and Kendall Col.,
Box 289
Huntsville, Alabama
Furniture ready to assemble; a catalogue gives prices

Superintendent of Documents
Government Printing Office
Washington, D. C. 20402

An up-to-date listing of government publications relating to carpentry, wood working and house maintenance is available without charge.

Better Homes and Gardens Handy Plan Service
1716 Locust Avenue
Des Moines, Iowa

Craft Patterns
North Avenue and RR 83
Elmhurst, Illinois

Craftsplans
1322 S. Wabash Avenue
Chicago 5, Illinois

American Plywood Association
119 A Street
Tacoma 2, Washington

U-Bild Enterprises
15155 Saticoy Street
Van Nuys, California

Popular Mechanics Press
200 E. Ontario Street
Chicago 11, Illinois

Specialties

Immerman and Sons
1924 Euclid Avenue
Cleveland 15, Ohio
Sukuragami craft

Benton-Kirby, Inc.
(414) 272-1690 445 North Broadway
Milwaukee, Wisconsin 53202

Gift shop supplies, activity program ideas — window sill planters, kits, large print song sheets with music, exercising games, reading magnifiers, etc.

Idea Exchange
Saverna Park, Maryland

Subscription $3.00 a year for four issues includes craft patterns, woodworking patterns, copper tooling, leather, paper crafts, rug designs, weaving, pottery, party decorations, knitting and braiding, useful and practical.

Complete Art Activities Almanac $3.50
Art Education Alumni
Wayne University
100 West Kirby Avenue
Detroit 2, Michigan

For dozens of patterns and step-by-step procedures in crafts, many of which can be used for handicapped people; pictures are easy to copy and simple directions in how-to-do wire figures, embroidery, soap carving, holiday decoration ideas, etc.

Fad-of-the-Month Club
Decorah, Iowa
Crafts come in the mail from the club with a different craft hobby
each month.

Western Pine Association
510 Yeon Building
Portland, Oregon
For wood carving
A linoleum paste, Grip Tite,® will work on tins, wooden boxes,
paper or linoleum; it is purchased where ceramic tile is sold.

Games

Candler's Bingo King
P.O. Box 1178
Englewood, Colorado 80110
#400 type card at 43¢ each for bingo with "seethru" plastic shutters

Mansfield-Zesiger Mfg. Co.
Cuyahoga Falls, Ohio
Portable bowling game, pins hang on a rod and flip over, very
popular game; $9.95 postpaid, includes one ball and one score pad;
extra balls are $1.50 and extra score pads 15¢.

Black Importing Co.
Richmond, Virginia
German roulette $2.00

Masenfield Bros. Inc.
Central Falls, R. I.
Bull's eye target game, styrofoam ball is thrown at plastic pointed pins
on target, for bed patients.

J. B. Birchall
2520 Glenwood
Rockford, Illinois 61103
Egyptian checkers in combination of checkers and Chinese checkers
with small blocks $13.90 a dozen.

Clubs, Discussion Groups, Pen Pals

The Federation of Aged People's Clubs in Japan would like
to exchange correspondence with senior groups in this country.
The address is, The Federation of Aged People's Clubs in Hyogo
Prefecture, C% Shakei Jigyo Kaikan, Nakayamate-dori 2-chome,
Ikuta-Ku, Kobe, Japan.

Grandmother Clubs of America; information is available by writing the National Headquarters of the Club, 203 North Wabash Avenue, Chicago 1, Illinois.

News discussion classes can be centered around weekly new sheets mailed each week to the Home; small size and easy to handle, large print, with questions; about 25¢ a semester; (fourth to sixth grade may be suitable). **Weekly Reader,** American Education Center, Wesleyan University Press, Inc., Columbus, Ohio, 43216.

Subscriptions to **Yankee,** an old-fashioned magazine from out of the past published in Dublin, New Hampshire, 03144, are $3.00 a year. Articles on the sinking of the **Titanic,** homes of our forefathers, stories by old-time sea captains, a woman who as a little girl posed for the illustrator of the Louisa Mae Alcott books, an interview with Robert Frost's daughter, fiction with old-time plots, beautiful colored photography, fascinating ads for items forgotten by anyone but the oldsters.

For the Visually Handicapped

The Christian Magnifier, a magazine in magnified print, is published by the Lutheran Braille Evangelism Association, $1.00 a year, the address, The Christian Magnifier, 902 Hennepin Avenue, Minneapolis, Minnesota.

Selected Hymns in church hymnals ($2.00) is printed in large type, published by the Augsburg Publishing House, 426 South Fifth Street, Minneapolis, 15, Minnesota 55415.

V and K Books, songbooks with half an inch high letters, no music, are obtained from Box 123, Madelia, Minnesota, $1.00 per book (1-20 copies), 90¢ per book (21-39 copies), 85¢ per book (40 or more copies), plus postage.

Also, "**Let's Sing Songbooks**" with the same large type, no music: Franciscan Sisters, St. Otto Home, Little Falls, Minnesota, 85¢ and postage.

Copies of the **Reader's Digest** are available in giant type, letters two and half times the size of those in the regular edition (¼" high); the volume size is 11" x 16". The new edition has been made possible by Xerox Corporation's process; machines will enlarge and print documents of all descriptions for about 14¢ a page. The regular edition of the **Digest** is microfilmed; the new edition's price is $4.50 a month or $25.65 for six months. Checks should be made out to Xerox Corporation. Full information may be obtained by writing to Xerox Corporation, PO Box 3300, Grand Central Station, New York, New York. A single copy comes in two volumes, no advertisements, and could be used by many residents.

A blind man may work on a "hobby knit loom" operated by one hand from Handcrafters, Waupun, Wisconsin; the loom is attached to a table edge, sells from $7.95; a ball of wool yarn is 50¢; free catalogues of supplies are available for rehabilitation purposes.

Special cards and games are available from American Foundation for the Blind, Inc., 15 West 16th Street, New York 11, N.Y. All prices include shipping costs. (The list follows.)

This nonprofit mail order service provides special devices, which in one way or another solves or reduces the problems resulting from blindness. Attention should be paid to the needs of the newly blind, as well as people in Homes who have developed experienced techniques to the problems of the partially sighted, as well as to those totally blind.

The Foundation encourages referrals on problems for which there does not seem to be a solution to be submitted to Special Services, which is often able to suggest a special device to be used by the visually handicapped.

French Chess Set. Raised and lowered squares and metal pegs to hold the pieces in place; colors have "flats" sanded on the white, $3.50.

Plastic checker board with men, 85¢.

Chinese Checkers. Wood-framed checker-board, with different shaped wooden checker men, $3.55.

Cribbage Boards. Holes are marked with grommets for easy location. Brass markers are in enclosure in rear, $2.60.

Imma Whiz. A mathematical bingo game; twenty-four cards carry six problems in multiplication and division; a deck of numbered cards is shuffled and the numbers called off one by one. When the number is the answer to a problem on a player's card, he makes note of it; cards in Braille and ink print, $1.45.

Brailled Dominoes. Made of molded black plastic with very prominent dots, $2.65.

Brailled Bicycle® Cards (bridge only). Standard deck with Braille dots. Markings at corners, 60¢.

Plastic Braillard Cards. Sturdier than Bicycle, solid plastic, durable dots, washable, $2.90.

Plastic Brailled Pinochle Cards.

Jumbo Cards. Playing cards with oversized symbols and numbers, for those with impaired vision.

Rook. This popular card game has been Brailled, $1.55.

Parcheesi. Ink print squares are replaced by holes into which the men (four different shapes) fit. Oversized dice read by touch, $2.70.

Bingo. Plastic board, depressions at the bottom, numbers appear in Braille. Wooden markers.

Scrabble®. Along the left edge, Braille characters showing the letter and its value. Board has ink print markings as well as Braille; also, built-in turning device. Tiles and tile racks mounted in separate tubular container used to shuffle the tiles; racks have built-in scoring devices like cribbage. Instructions in Braille and ink print as well as plastic Braille card giving value and distribution of the tiles, $5.50.

Anagram Tiles. Scrabble board makes a rack for setting up words. The plastic list included with Scrabble gives the distribution letters. Separate sets of the tiles combined with those in Scrabble, $1.50.

Sewing Aids For The Blind

Handy Magnet. Magnet with handle for picking up pins, small nails and other iron or steel objects, 25¢.

Hem Gauge. Marks hems with pins accurately and quickly; when a hinged arm is pressed against the skirt, it crimps the cloth and supplies a metal guide into which the pins are inserted, $1.60.

Redi-Thred® Needles. Formed to carry a wire loop permanently secured to the needle eye. The wire loop, which is easy to thread, trails behind the needle so it will not spread warp or woof; locks even nylon thread in place, 20¢.

Wire Loop Threaders. Thread can be placed in loop and drawn through eye of needle. Free.

Other Aids

Other aids include geographical maps and globes; mathematical aids; slates, compasses, protractors and slide rules; coin changers, fire extinguishers, key keepers, pipe and cigarette lighters, pocket ashtrays, calendars and pinch purses.

Tellatouch. A device for communication between a sighted or blind person and a deaf-blind person who reads Braille. No training or special skill required; weighs three pounds; not a typewriter or a Braille writer, $42.50.

Hobbyists with tape records: Blind residents may become members of the Voicespondence Club International, Noel, Virginia; $4.00 for annual dues; memberships are world wide. Hobbyists with tape recorders are listed with their special interests in code, special interests which they may share with new friends; a nonprofit organization, members exchange tapes which they have made.

A Lutheran organization publishes and distributes Christian literature for the blind and visually handicapped: Lutheran Braille Evangelism Association, 1619 Portland Avenue South, Minneapolis, Minnesota, 55404.

Jarts® is an outdoor game made of heavy metal and plastic; tossed like horseshoes, the "jarts" stand up in the ground landing inside the target ring. Two or more may play, the leader's voice directing players as to where to throw the jarts. Replacements are available; World Wide Games, Radnor Road, Delaware, Ohio 43015.

For the Musically Inclined

Rhythm band instruments are available from music stores: jingle hammers, humanatones, kazoos (clarinet, trombone, cornet) sand blocks, rhythm sticks; a can of Sansprae ($1.65) should be used as an antiseptic for instruments which are shared.

Square Dance Records

World of Fun Records. Square dance records: Cokesbury, 1661 Northwest Highway, Park Ridge, Illinois, 60068; each record is $2.00; 78 rpm; an instruction sheet is included with each record.

Instruction book for the dances is $2.00.

Record M101 Hungarian, Swiss, Lithuanian, Austrian.

M102 Irish, Danish, "Captain Jinks."

M103 "Irish Washwoman."

M104 Red River Valley (USA), "Sicillian Circle," "Camptown Races" (USA), "Pop Goes the Weasel" (USA) and a variety of other records from many other ethnic groups.

Suggestions for rhythm band records might include:

"Rhythmic Activities," Vol. 1, Primary Grades, RCA Victor.

"Rhythm Band Album for Elementary Grades." RCA Victor.

And the following books:

"Melody, Rhythm, and Harmony" (familiar songs). Teacher's book, $1.85. Student's book, 85¢.

"Miniatures for Rhythm Band," Summerfield, $1.80.

"Reading in Rhythm," Strouse, Student Book, 40¢.

"Rhythm Is Fun," Beginner's Manual, instruments described, how to play, etc., $1.25.

"Rhythm Band Series," Votow-Laederach, Mennheimer, $1.25.

"Rhythm and Song," Elementary School Rhythms, Day, $1.50.

"American Singer," First Grade Teacher's Manual, American Book Company.

"Music in Early Childhood," Silver-Burdette Company.

"Rhythm Band Music" (piano), Edna Everett Beckley-Cardy Company.

At most music stores: jingle hammer, 90¢; humanatones, 15¢; clarinet kazoo, 70¢; trombone kazoo, 75¢; coronet kazoo, 75¢; sand block, $1.45; rhythm sticks, 20¢; one can Sansprae® (disinfectant for the mouth instruments to be used each time), $1.65.

BOUNCING BALL SING-ALONGS. The old-fashioned bouncing ball sing-along films, such as were featured in movie theatres are available: write Twymwn Films, 329 Salem Avenue, Dayton, Ohio, for information. In black and white: "Let's All Sing Together," "Sing, America," "Sing and Be Happy". And in color: "Comin' Round the Mountain"; "Base Brawl"; "Spring Song," "Strolling Thru the Park."

For the Nature Lover

1. BARTON, ROGER: *How to Watch Birds*. New York, McGray, 1955, 229 pages. Written by a birdwatcher who has made a study of his hobby. $1.95.

2. CAMPBELL, SAM: *Nature's Messages: A Book of Wilderness Wisdom*. Chicago, Rand McNally, 1952, 221 pages. The author describes the seasons as they come to his home in the Nicolet National Forest in Wisconsin. $2.95

3. Cornell Laboratory of Ornithology; *Field Guide to Bird Songs of Eastern and Central North America*. Boston, Houghton and Mifflin, 1959, $10.95. A series of long-playing records are produced by the Cornell Laboratory of Ornithology. $10.95. Orders should be sent directly to Invoice Processing, Houghton Mifflin Company, Wayside Road, Burlington, Massachusetts.

4. DOOLE, LOUISE EVANS:*Herb and Garden Ideas*. New York, Sterling, 1964, 108 pages. The title does not indicate the range of project ideas which are described here. "Gardens from Leftovers" and "Indoor Gardens" should have great appeal. $2.95.

5. EIFERT, VIRGINIA: *Men, Birds and Adventure; the Thrilling Story of the Discovery of American Birds*. New York, Houghton and Mifflin, 1962, 273 pages, $3.50.

6. HICKEY, JOSEPH J.: *A Guide to Bird Watching*, Boston and New York, Doubleday Anchor Book (N30) 1963, 262 pages. $1.25.

7. McELROY, THOMAS P.: *New Handbook of Attracting Birds*. New York, Knopf, 1960, 163 pages. $4.00.

8. PETERSON, ROGER TORY, AND JAMES FISHER: *Wild America*. Cambridge Massachusetts, Houghton and Mifflin, 1963 (Sentry 35), 434 pages. Stimulating reading on nature subjects. Print is clear and the book is easy to hold. $2.85.

9. SCHUTZ, WALTER E.: *Bird Watching, Housing and Feeding*. Milwaukee, Bruce, 1963, 168 pages. $3.75.

10. WETMORE, ALEXANDER AND OTHERS: *Song and Garden Birds of North America*. Washington, National Geographic Society, 1964, 400 pages. Records are included. This is a beautiful book to examine and enjoy; however, it is heavy to hold. The recordings which are tucked into the back of the book are a joy. Suggest as a gift or memorial. $11.95.

For other listings of books on nature, the booklist, *Profiles of*

Nature, may be requested from the Wisconsin Free Library Commission, P.O. Box 1437, Madison, Wisconsin. Books may be available from other state commissions if the Home has no access to a public library.

Many inexpensive books (from 35¢ to $1.00) on tropical fish, cats, plants and garden, birds and dogs are available from T. F. H. Publications, Inc. 245-247 Cornelison Avenue, P.O. Box 33, Jersey City 2, N. J.

For Ambulatory Residents

Residents read the lines from script typed in capitals; play rehearsals are scheduled with the daily program on the bulletin board.

The following companies furnish catalogues of plays and dialogues suitable for oldsters' productions with limited props, sets and costumes and with homey, folksy, old-time themes:

Beckley-Cardy Company
1900 North Narragansett
Chicago, Illinois 60639

Paine Publishing Company
34 N. Jefferson Street
Dayton 1, Ohio

(**Snappy Comedies** [from which "A Husband for Harriet" was very popular]).

Eldridge Company
Franklin, Ohio

The Northwest Press
315 Fifth Avenue South
Minneapolis, Minnesota

T. S. Dennison and Company
623 South Wabash Avenue
Chicago, Illinois

For the Dramatic Club, "Pioneers in Petticoats," Nelly McCaslin has thirteen short plays "based on the colorful personalities of some of our nation's heroines." For resident talent programs and simple productions: "Pioneers in Petticoats," Row Peterson, Evanston, Ill. $2.00.

Catchy Loose-leaf Play Series are six cents a copy from Willis N. Bugbie Co., Syracuse, N.Y.

Further Addresses for Running the Program

The state occupational therapy associations are in the process of locating all registered occupational therapists throughout their respective state, listing therapists who are interested in returning to work full-time or part-time. By inquiring of some certified occupational therapist in the community, the state placement chairman may be located.

Where to Sell Handicrafts, published by Charles Brandford, 1951, 208 Union Street, Newton Centre, 59 Massachusetts, may be useful in disposing of crafts.

Addresses of Agencies and Their Needs

Missionary Association, 1425 North Prospect Avenue, Milwaukee, Wisconsin, 53202, can use stuffed toys for missions, quilts, worn sheets and pillow cases torn into bandages in all sizes 1″, 1½″, 2″ or 3″ wide, and five yards long, babies' layettes, children's clothing, mittens, socks, caps and scarves; altar linens; leper bandages knitted of new or old wool of different color odds and ends. (Use medium needles, knit in garter stitch 3″ wide, 1½ yards long, 16 stitches regular wool or 18 fine wool.) They would also like leper scarves 18″ x 60″.

Catholic Maternity Institute, 417 E. Palace Avenue, Santa Fe, New Mexico can use pot holders, rosaries, baby clothes.

Bethesda Lutheran Home, 700 Hoffman Drive, Watertown, Wisconsin 53094 can use quilts, washable, 63″ x 90″ machine sewed, bibs and favors.

Lutheran Children's Friend Society, 8138 Harwood Avenue, Wauwatosa, Wisconsin 53213 can use pot holders and covered hangers.

Sister Christens, Holy Child School, Box 297 B, Moore, Okla. collects cancelled stamps.

Genevieve Feyen, Pax Christi, 708 Avenue I, Greenwood, Miss. staffs a medical dispensary that "treats people with headaches to the most complicated diseases. Any assistance from one bandage to pictures for rooms, will be put to use immediately . . ."

Agencies to Which You May Refer

Jewish Federation of Omaha
101 North 20th Street
Omaha 2, Nebraska
Film and film strip library on aging, catalogue; $2.00-$7.00 rental on films.

New York State Office for the Aging
Executive Dept.
112 State Street
Albany, New York 12201
Surveys of state and community programs for aging.

Selected References on Aging
Dept. of Health, Education and Welfare
Washington, D. C. 20201

National Recreation and Park Association
8 West Eighth Street
New York, New York 10011
Guide to books on recreation. 25¢.

A Program of Recreation for the Homebound Adult

Morton Thompson, Ed.D.
Consultant, Recreation for the Ill and Handicapped
A manual based on recommendations of the Office of Vocational Rehabilitation Project.

Proud Years, a 16 mm sound black and white, 28 min. 1956. Produced by Columbia University Mass Communication Center in collaboration with the Medical Directors of the Home for Aged and Infirm Hebrews of N.Y., Charles Pfizer and Company; good training film.

CLASSIFICATION CHART
OF ACTIVITIES ACCORDING TO HANDICAPS

Early in the working stages of the book, this type of chart was planned for quick referral of suitable activities for the handicaps discussed in the book.

For instance, the leader beset with difficulties in finding activities for wheelchair patients in the dayroom needs an on-the-spot activity. What can be done for sixteen people with a variety of handicaps? She looks at the chart under "Wheelchair" and finds what wheelchair residents are able to do, looks under the column also for "Two or More" and finds a variety of activities for a group of wheelchair patients. She notices, too, that many of these patients have visual handicaps, and under that column finds page numbers for activities possible for this additional handicap.

On the wards she may need activity for "Bed" patients; or in good weather deciding to take residents outside, she looks under "Outdoors" for suitable activities evaluated in the chart.

The chart is an Index in that every activity in the book is listed except the Part III material.

ACTIVITIES INDEX CHART

APHASIC	VISUALLY HANDICAPPED	SENESCENT	BED	WHEELCHAIR	SEMI-AMBULANT	INDEPENDENT	2 OR MORE	1 PERSON	INDOORS	OUTDOORS	
×				×	×	×	×	×	×		Building, Ice Shanty, 223
×				×	×		×		×		Bumper Pool, 147
×				×	×		×		×	×	Bunco, 132
×	×			×	×		×		×	×	Button, Button, 141
×	×			×	×		×		×	×	Buttoning (stunt), 140
×			×	×	×	×		×	×	×	Carnation (Kleenex), 228
×				×	×	×		×	×	×	Carpentry Novelties, 226
×				×	×	×		×	×	×	Carving Wood, 225
×	×			×	×		×		×	×	Cane Race (stunt), 140
×				×	×	×		×	×		Ceramics, 207
×				×	×		×		×	×	Charades (stunt), 142
×			×	×	×		×		×	×	Charge Account, 132
×	×		×	×	×		×		×	×	Checker Tournament, 112, 145
×				×	×	×		×	×		Cheese Board, 221
×			×	×	×	×		×	×		Christmas Crafts, 211
×			×	×	×	×		×	×		Christmas Tree, 212
	×			×	×		×		×	×	Chit and Chat, 163
				×	×		×		×	×	Choral Reading, 183
×	×			×	×		×		×	×	Clubs, 150
×			×	×	×			×	×		Collections, 117
×			×	×	×	×		×	×	×	Container (craft), 205
	×	×		×	×		×		×	×	Community Sings, 170
×			×	×	×		×	×	×	×	Concentration Party, 113
			×	×	×		×		×	×	Conversation, 163, 165
×				×	×	×	×		×		Cooking Class, 192

APHASIC	VISUALLY HANDICAPPED	SENESCENT	BED	WHEELCHAIR	SEMI-AMBULANT	INDEPENDENT	2 OR MORE	1 PERSON	INDOORS	OUTDOORS	
×	×	×	×	×	×	×	×	×	×	×	Hobby List, 149, 150
×				×	×		×		×	×	Hobby Show, 149
×			×	×	×	×		×	×	×	Hooked Yarn, 233
×	×			×	×		×		×	×	Horse Racing, 114
×	×	×		×	×		×		×	×	Horseshoes, 147
×			×	×	×	×		×	×	×	Huck Toweling, 232
			×	×	×	×	×	×	×	×	Icebreakers, 110
	×		×	×	×		×		×	×	Identifying (stunt), 142
			×	×		×		×			I Doubt You, 130
			×	×		×		×			Indian, 134
×	×		×	×	×		×		×	×	Investment Club, 156
×	×		×	×	×	×	×	×	×	×	Isometric Exercises, 126
	×			×	×		×		×	×	I've Got a Secret, 145
×				×	×		×			×	Jarts, 148
×			×	×	×	×		×	×	×	Jeweled Trinket Box, 214
×				×	×	×		×	×		Knitting on Custom Loom, 232
×	×			×	×		×		×	×	Knocking Off Hats, (stunt), 138
	×			×	×		×		×	×	League of Women Voters, 158
×			×	×	×	×		×	×	×	Leather Work, 207
					×		×		×	×	Left Handed Mixer (stunt), 255
	×			×	×		×		×	×	Literary Club, 157
×	×	×	×	×	×	×		×	×	×	Macaroni Wreath, 212
					×		×		×	×	Man in the Moon (stunt), 258
×				×	×	×		×	×		Marble Jewelry, 207
×	×			×	×		×		×	×	Marshmallow Eating (stunt), 140

APHASIC	VISUALLY HANDICAPPED	SENESCENT	BED	WHEELCHAIR	SEMI-AMBULANT	INDEPENDENT	2 OR MORE	1 PERSON	INDOORS	OUTDOORS	
×					×		×		×	×	Miniature Golf, 249
×	×		×	×	×	×		×	×	×	Mosaic Tile, 237
		×	×	×	×		×		×	×	Mounting Pictures, 206, 210
×		×	×	×	×		×		×		Movies, 175
×	×		×	×	×		×		×	×	Music Appreciation Class, 171
×	×	×	×	×	×		×		×	×	Music from the Community, 172
×	×			×	×	×	×	×	×	×	Musicians, 172
			×	×	×		×		×	×	News Discussion, 168
×					×		×		×	×	On the Spot (stunt), 258
×				×	×		×		×		O Pshaw (game), 133
	×		×	×	×		×	×	×	×	Oral Quizzes, 306
×			×	×	×	×		×	×	×	Paper Rose, 228
×					×		×		×	×	Paper Bags (stunt), 258
×					×		×		×	×	Passing the Egg (stunt), 247
	×			×	×		×		×	×	Password, 144
×				×	×		×		×	×	Patch Race (stunt), 140
×			×	×	×	×		×	×		Pen Pals, 117
×	×		×	×	×		×		×	×	Picking Apples (stunt), 140
×				×	×	×				×	Picnic Program, 246
×	×	×		×	×		×			×	Picnics, 244
×				×	×	×		×	×		Picture Frames, 223
×				×	×	×		×	×	×	Pictures, Gauzed, Sprayed, 206
×				×	×		×		×		Pig (game), 134
×			×	×	×	×		×	×	×	Pillows, Lap Robes, 204
×	×	×		×	×	×	×	×	×		Pin Ball, 147

APHASIC	VISUALLY HANDICAPPED	SENESCENT	BED	WHEELCHAIR	SEMI-AMBULANT	INDEPENDENT	2 OR MORE	1 PERSON	INDOORS	OUTDOORS	
×	×		×	×	×	×		×	×	×	Salvage Material Crafts, 204
×			×	×	×	×		×	×	×	Satin Sachet, 230
×			×	×	×	×		×	×	×	Seed Mosaics, 234
×			×	×	×	×	×	×	×	×	Sewing Projects, 112,197,201,226
×		×	×	×	×	×		×	×	×	Sewing Rags for Rugs, 232
×	×		×	×	×	×	×	×	×	×	Shaggy Rug, 123
×				×	×		×		×	×	Shaving (stunt), 139
×				×	×		×		×	×	Shoes, Mixing (stunt), 247
					×		×		×	×	Signature Hunt (stunt), 257
×				×	×		×		×	×	Singo, 174
×					×		×		×	×	Skeleton Name (stunt), 258
×		×	×	×	×	×	×	×	×	×	Sketching Class, 208
					×		×		×	×	Skit, 251
×	×	×			×		×		×	×	Slipper Kick (stunt), 247
	×	×		×	×		×		×	×	Social Clubs, 150, 156-161
	×	×		×	×		×		×	×	Socializing, 155
	×			×	×		×		×	×	Spelldowns, 143
	×			×	×		×		×	×	Sportsmen's Club, 158
	×			×	×			×	×	×	Story Telling Hour, 158
×	×	×	×	×	×	×	×	×	×	×	Stuffing Animals, Dolls, 201
×	×			×	×		×		×	×	Stunts, Wheelchairs, 138
×		×	×	×	×		×		×	×	Suction Darts, 112
×	×	×		×	×		×		×	×	Supper Club, 158
×		×		×	×	×	×		×		Table Shuffleboard, 147
	×			×	×		×		×	×	Talent Shows, 172, 250

APHASIC	VISUALLY HANDICAPPED	SENESCENT	BED	WHEELCHAIR	SEMI-AMBULANT	INDEPENDENT	2 OR MORE	1 PERSON	INDOORS	OUTDOORS	
	×			×	×		×		×	×	What's My Line?, 144
					×		×		×	×	What's Your Name? (stunt), 258
				×	×		×		×	×	What You're Doing (stunt), 255
×				×	×		×			×	Wheelchair Croquet, 148
×	×	×		×			×		×	×	Wheelchair Square Dance, 168
×				×	×		×		×	×	Whirley Bird, 147
×			×	×	×	×		×	×	×	Whittling, 225
×	×	×		×	×	×		×	×	×	Work in the Home, 189
×				×	×		×		×	×	Wrapping Packages (stunt), 138
×			×	×	×	×		×	×	×	Writing, Local Paper, 181
×			×	×	×	×		×	×	×	Written Quizzes, 332